Mind Games

The Aging Brain and How to Keep it Healthy

To Glenn, my father, the ubiquitous thaumaturgist
and
To Keith, for his unwavering devotion and support.
Kathleen

To my husband Lew, daughter Shara, and mother Virginia.
and
To God, through whom all things are possible.
Kathryn

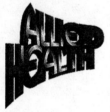

Mind Games

The Aging Brain and How to Keep it Healthy

Kathryn C. Wetzel, PhD
Kathleen M. Harmeyer, MS

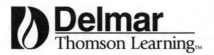

Africa • Australia • Canada • Denmark • Japan • Mexico • New Zealand • Philippines
Puerto Rico • Singapore • Spain • United Kingdom • United States

Notice to the Reader

Publisher does not warrant or guarantee any of the products described herein or perform any independent analysis in connection with any of the product information contained herein. Publisher does not assume, and expressly disclaims, any obligation to obtain and include information other than that provided to it by the manufacturer.

The reader is expressly warned to consider and adopt all safety precautions that might be indicated by the activities herein and to avoid all potential hazards. By following the instructions contained herein, the reader willingly assumes all risks in connection with such instructions.

The publisher makes no representation or warranties of any kind, including but not limited to the warranties of fitness for a particular purpose or merchantability, nor are any such representations implied with respect to the material set forth herein, and the publisher takes no responsibility with respect to such material. The publisher shall not be liable for any special, consequential, or exemplary damages resulting, in whole or part, from the reader's use of, or reliance upon, this material.

Delmar Staff:

Health Care Publishing Director: William Brottmiller
Product Development Manager: Marion S. Waldman
Developmental Editor: Maria Perretta
Executive Marketing Manager: Dawn F. Gerrain
Channel Manager: Jayme McRee
Project Editor: Christopher C. Leonard
Production Coordinator: James Zayicek
Art/Design Coordinator: Jay Purcell
Cover Design: Jay Purcell

For more information, contact Delmar, 3 Columbia Circle, P.O. Box 15015, Albany, NY 12212–0515; or find us on the Web at http://www.delmar.com

Library of Congress Cataloging-in-Publication Data

Wetzel, Kathryn C.
    Mind games: the aging brain and how to keep it healthy / by Kathryn C. Wetzel and Kathleen M. Harmeyer.
        p.   cm.
    Includes bibliographical references and index.
    ISBN 0-7668-1280-4
    1. Cognition—Age factors. 2. Memory—Age factors. 3. Human information processing—Age factors. 4. Aging—Psychological aspects. I. Harmeyer, Kathleen M. II. Title.
  BF724.55.C63 W48   1999
  155.67'13—dc21   99-39159

Contents

Note:
According to D. Warner Schaie, while minor memory lapses and some slowing of mental processes are normal aspects of the aging process, in some people they could be early signs of depression or dementia. Individuals who have serious concerns about memory losses or losses in other cognitive skills should seek professional help from a psychologist or psychiatrist.

PREFACE

Attention All People Over 40!

WHY YOU SHOULD READ THIS BOOK

Regardless of your age, have you ever experienced what may be affectionately described as "senior moments?" For example, have you

- Checked three or four times to make sure that the same appliance is turned off before you leave home?
- Tried to use a word in your conversation that you *know* you know but cannot recall?
- Walked up and down the parking lot looking for your car, with the grocery sacker tagging along behind?
- Forgotten someone's name you just met, even though you were rehearsing it while you were walking away?
- Had someone tell you that you do not correctly remember what he or she told you?

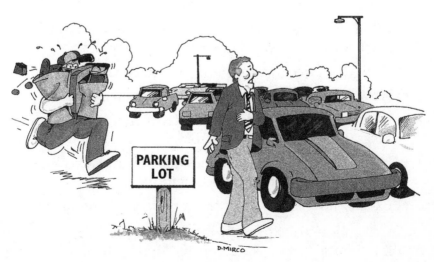

Or, you may be apprehensive of your ability to adapt to new situations. Are you concerned that rusty brain cells may prevent you from successfully

- Moving to a new home or city?
- Joining a special-interest group to meet new friends?
- Earning a degree or enrolling in a continuing-education course?
- Applying for a new job?
- Managing your business and/or life?

Well, if you answered "yes" to any of these questions or have similar worries in your life, it's not hopeless. This book is just what you need. It explains why these "senior moments" occur and how you can take charge of your mental agility. You just need to exercise those brain cells to become more mentally alert and agile. Athletes train and maintain their bodies in peak operating condition. You need to train and maintain your brain. Keep in mind—pardon the pun—that this text is not just a book to improve your memory. It is designed to give you pertinent information regarding the quality of your life.

You'll find information such as

- Why certain aspects of your thinking processes are more finely tuned than others
- What the latest learning theory is, explained in layperson's terms, based on recent brain research
- How diet affects your memory and capacity to think
- How physical exercise relates to mental exercise
- Why research regarding the effects of aging is, in many cases, seemingly contradictory
- How the suggested strategies, games, and activities can increase your thinking and memory capacity
- Exactly how to regain and maintain your mental agility

We'll guide you through the learning-style preferences and the mental-processing modes that will promote the most mental growth for you. You'll be able to apply these learning techniques and strategies to all aspects of your life—excelling at work, returning to school, learning a hobby, overcoming drastic changes in your health, and more. This book is designed for middle-aged adults, senior citizens, healthcare professionals, and home caregivers.

THE RESEARCH BASIS

The Seattle Longitudinal Study, a program conducted for more than 40 years by K. Warner Schaie, PhD., an Evan Pugh Professor at Pennsylvania State University, charted the course of selected cognitive abilities as the study population aged. After noting the decline in mental acuity in elders, Schaie, along with Dr. Sherry Willis, instituted a five-hour training session with specific mental exercises. The exercises addressed inductive reasoning techniques and spatial relationship skills, among others. After that period, the majority of the people trained demonstrated that they had regained and could continue to maintain the same mental agility they had exhibited 14 years ago.

Based on Schaie's work, the results of comparable research, and our combined 47 years of teaching expertise, this text is designed to assist you in regaining and maintaining the mental agility you may have lost. It also will help you successfully pursue lifelong learning.

HOW TO USE THIS BOOK

Chapter 1 begins with a look at how you as an individual prefer to learn. Chapters 2 through 4 continue with a physical description of how the brain functions. You then examine the effects commonly associated with the aging process (Chapter 5) and then rapidly proceed to specific measures you easily can use to regain and maintain mental agility (Chapters 6 and 7). This text builds a concrete foundation by explaining the premise on which all of the learning and retention strategies are based.

If you are a sequential learner (one who starts at the beginning and performs each step along the way), you will progress through the chapters, and by the time you reach Chapter 6, you will fully understand the relevance of the games, exercises, projects, hobbies, and activities the text recommends. Nonsequential learners (those who look for a specific topic and start there) who skip directly to Chapter 6 will discover many references back to explanations in earlier chapters. As you become more interested in the material presented, you easily can refer back to the applicable foundation theory.

Whether you are a sequential or nonsequential learner, we strongly recommend that you eventually read all of the chapters to receive the full benefit of the information.

We present key concepts at the beginning of each chapter. After you identify a favored learning style, icons direct you to the appropriate learning activity. For example, numerous diagrams, photographs, and illustrations guide the learning for readers who have difficulty visualizing information from text. Inserts highlight special enrichment concepts and role-model experiences.

To support the text, we have set up a Web site with animations that are keyed to text explanations. Interactive games for mental exercises described in the text also are available on the Web. All of the exercises, games, and learning strategies directly affect specific areas of the brain and allow for growth and development of widely applicable learning and retention skills. You will find a supplement at the Web site with teaching strategies and ideas applicable for a classroom setting or discussion group. Visit www.mentalagility.com.

MIDDLE-AGED ADULTS, SENIOR CITIZENS, AND ELDERS

If you want to dust off your brain cells and fine-tune your thinking processes, you can practice these learning strategies anywhere at any time. You may initially read and practice the exercises and games included in this text at home, while at the hairdresser's or barber's, or even in bed before you go to sleep. However, after you understand the reasoning behind the techniques, you will begin applying them to situations independent from the book—while at work, driving, fishing, or shopping. If you practice these techniques, they *will* make a difference in your life and improve the quality of your lifestyle. You will feel in control again.

HEALTHCARE PROFESSIONALS AND HOME CAREGIVERS

This text supports a continuing-education class on assisting seniors to regain their mental acuity. The material is presented clearly in layperson's terminology, laced with humor and everyday application strategies. Students in the class will enjoy group discussions of their experiences. The exercises and activities in this book easily may be adapted to group activities.

For those of you who care for another person in the home, this book can help provide assistance in explaining the reasons for that person's apparent decline and in selecting activities to help reverse the process.

Healthcare professionals serving the elder population may use this text to supplement the daily routine of their elderly patients in group sessions. Some elderly patients may prefer to use the text on an individual basis instead of in a classroom setting. If your patients have physical complications and cannot read, you should read through the entire book prior to meeting with them about this topic. Explain Chapters 1 through 4 and help them with the tests on learning preferences in Chapter 1. It might help them to know many of the aspects of aging, such as why food doesn't seem to interest them as it used to. You'll find this information in Chapter 5. As the healthcare giver, you will need to evaluate your patient and choose appropriate exercises, games, and activities from all the chapters, but especially those in Chapters 4, 6, and 7.

SUMMARY

This book gives you proven techniques that will help rejuvenate the minds of those who perform the exercises. It is based on solid university research that produced stunning results. Humor is beneficial to mental health, so remember to have fun while you are doing these exercises.

> *"The intelligent man is one who has successfully fulfilled many accomplishments, and is yet willing to learn more."* — *Ed Parker*

ACKNOWLEDGEMENTS

A million thanks to our families who did everything else, while we wrote.

Special thanks to Tom Reppenhagen, Sharon Mulgrew and Myan Baker, for key contributions to the process. And to Rosemary Austin, who worked all the exercises.

Thanks to the people who helped with the publishing process, including our editors, Marlene Pratt, Maria Perretta; our art coordinator, Jay Purcell; and our production editor, Beth Brown. Thank you for supplying PET scans, Dr. Marcus Raichle and Dr. John Mazziotta. And to Nancy Klingsick who never said no. And to influential teachers, Colleen Pierre and Fran Lannon.

Thanks for graciously allowing us to photograph you: Glenn Austin, Rosemary Austin, Billie Ballard, Buddy Ballard, Debra Baze, Virginia Chestnut, Jesse Coon, Dorothy DiMaio, Marguerite Empie, Chuck Gibson, Jacque Gibson, Bob Gifford, Rita Gifford, Janet Harter, Khabir, Leo LaBorde, Gene McLane, Helen McLane, Victoria Mok, Sharon Mulgrew, Antonio Salazar, Bryan Umeki, Doris Waller and Brackston Yarborough who assisted with the photographs of Leo LaBorde.

Sincere thanks to our talented photographers, Amy Aldrich, Winfield Leitzer, and Henry Ortega. And for invaluable moral support, Carrol Spears, Aimee Martin, and Bobby May.

The Learning Styles of an Agile Mind

Discover How You Capture, Select and Store Information

KEY CONCEPTS

How We Capture Information
How Memories Are Made
Learning Styles
Learning Styles Investigation
Using Learning Style

INTRODUCTION

You are bombarded with information every waking moment. Once selected, some information passes from immediate memory—that is, what you can sense—into short-term or holding memory. Finally, a small amount of the original information makes it to permanent long-term memory. The final move to long-term memory is what we call *learning*. In this chapter, you will learn how information is captured, selected, and stored.

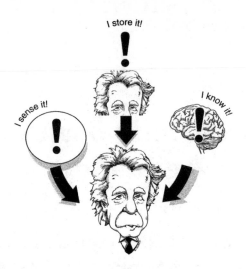

CAPTURING INFORMATION

You obtain information through your five senses: sight, hearing, touch, smell, and taste. Imagine yourself watching a television program about your favorite hobby. You see and hear the information. You receive this information in an auditory manner (you hear it) and visually (you see it). These delivery methods, using only two of your five senses, are how the majority of people believe information is taught and learned. The truth is that a great deal of information is conveyed to you through your other senses: smell, taste, and touch. *Olfactory* (smell) and *gustatory* (taste) sensations are more rarely used in formal learning activities than hearing and sight. However, people rely extensively on these senses in the home and at work (detecting smoke, gas leaks, cooking, and so on). You know the old adage, "The way to a man's heart is through his stomach!"

Your sense of touch also tells you a great deal about the world around you. You use it to check a child's temperature, the fineness of your handiwork, or the car's vibration. Your sense of touch is intricately involved in your *kinesthetic* (motor) skills with which you write, learn a new hobby, drive, get dressed, and many, many other physical activities. Some emotional information is communicated through touch, such as a gentle pat or a warm, loving hug.

MAKING MEMORIES

Imagine yourself at an elegant party. People are talking, dishes and utensils are clinking, and music is playing softly in the background. Soft candlelight illuminates silk-covered furnishings while the aroma of dinner fills the air.

All of these impressions saturate your five senses, which trans-fer as much information as they can to the brain via what is called the *sensory store.* These fleeting sensations remain for only a few milliseconds before the majority of the sensations are lost and only a small subset is passed on to *short-term,* or working, *memory* (STM). The information is lost within 15 to 30 seconds if not selected for closer consideration. If you were not paying attention to a conversation, you could reconstruct a recent comment if asked within this 15 to 30 second window. However, after this brief interval of time, you must begin to organize and rehearse the information you want to store in *long-term memory* (LTM). The process of learning new information does not stop when we go to sleep. Recent research indicates that sleep is essential to the formation and efficient storage of memories. As we sleep, the brain appears to replay the activities of the day, reactivating old and activating new brain cell connections. With proper encoding and retrieval strategies, information that is stored in LTM is considered relatively permanent because it can be recalled years later.[1]

> *Sleep is essential to the formation and efficient storage of memories.*

The overwhelming mode of human communication is a mix of verbal and visual information. Figure 1-1 shows brain images, which demonstrate the different parts of the brain that are active when listening to words and looking at words.

Notice that if material is presented orally, the brain reacts as shown in Figure 1-1a, whereas if material is presented visually, the brain reacts as shown in Figure 1-1b.

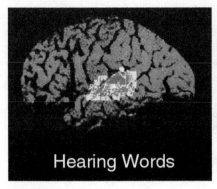
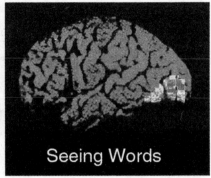

Hearing Words   Seeing Words

Figure I-la Hearing Words   **Figure I-lb** Seeing Words
Figure   Figure

LEARNING STYLES

auditory learner—one who prefers to listen to new
information.

visual learner—one who prefers to see new
information.

kinesthetic learner—one who prefers to practice
new information.

Some people prefer to listen to new information and are
called *auditory learners,* whereas others prefer to see the new
information and are described as *visual learners.* If you listen
primarily to words on the radio, on television, and in conversation, the sections of your brain that are activated
(Hearing Words, as shown in Figure 1-1a) become stronger,
just as the specific muscles a body builder exercises grow
stronger. Similarly, when you see the words, the sections of
your brain that are activated (Seeing Words, as shown in
Figure 1-1b) become stronger.

Still other people prefer to write down new information
or to practice a new skill and are classified as *kinesthetic
learners.* You may prefer to learn using only one of the auditory, visual, and kinesthetic techniques. The white areas in
Figure 1-2 show the regions of brain activity for auditory, vi-

sual, and kinesthetic (motor) stimulation. Different areas of the brain respond to different delivery formats.

In this text, you will see several PET scans, so a description of the technique might be helpful. A radioactive substance with a short half-life is injected into the bloodstream using glucose as the carrier. The radioactivity allows external monitoring of the metabolism of the brain. Sensors around the volunteer's head monitor the radioactivity. Computers convert the information into two-dimensional images. The more active an area of the brain, the more glucose it uses, and the brighter the color. In black-and-white pictures, the more active areas show up whiter. The other areas of the brain are not dormant. They are simply not as active.

Begin to notice how you prefer to have information presented. You may prefer to use a combination of auditory, visual, and kinesthetic (motor) methods. For example, you might repeat a written list aloud while marking items off on your fingers. Do you want someone to give you written directions rather than to tell you how to get somewhere? Would you rather listen to a book on tape than to read a book? Do you move or shift around, adjust your tie, twirl your hair, or otherwise "fidget" when concentrating? Do you believe you are an auditory, visual, or kinesthetic learner?

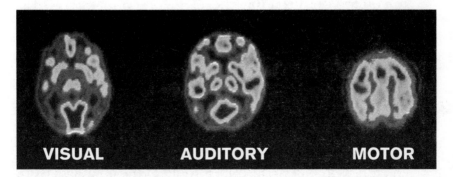

Figure 1-2   Brain activity for visual, auditory, and kinesthetic stimulation

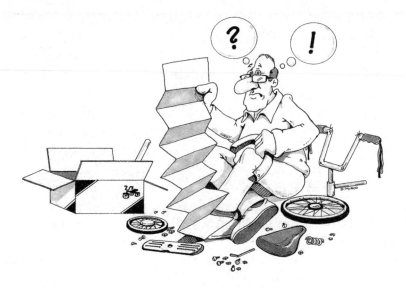

Suppose for a moment that you have purchased a piece of furniture or a toy that requires assembly.

Visualize the contents of the box. Usually there are parts and a set of directions. How do you attack this problem? Do you

1. Read the directions thoroughly and/or study each diagram before beginning assembly?

2. Read the directions aloud or ask someone to read them to you as you put it together?

3. Look at the parts, ignore the directions, and start to assemble it right away?

If you selected number 1 as the action you would most likely take, it is conceivable that you have a visual learning preference. An auditory learner may prefer to hear the instructions or speak them aloud—number 2. The kinesthetic learner knows how the pieces fit together and jumps right in—number 3.

The following table describes some of the characteristics typically displayed by the three types of learners. Take just a few minutes, using your own self-awareness and the table. Try to decide whether you would describe yourself as an auditory, visual, or kinesthetic learner.

Auditory Learner	**Visual Learner**	**Kinesthetic Learner**
Often described as a talker	Watches the faces of talkers	Likes to move around a lot
Quickly learns words to songs	Can "see" where something is located	Likes to touch things
May reverse b-d or p-q when writing	May misinterpret spoken words	Does not like to read directions
May not enjoy writing	Would rather write things down	Would rather write things down
Keeps poor track of time	May have a good sense of color	Lives in the present. Poor sense of time
May get lost in new territory	Mind may wander while listening to others talk	Restless. Paces while on the phone
May not be adept at reading body language or facial expressions	Likes symmetry	Learns best by doing
Favorite phrases: "That sounds good." "I hear you."	Favorite phrases: "I see." "I get the picture."	Favorite phrases: "I feel ..." "I need to get a handle on ..."

So what did you decide? Are you primarily an auditory, visual, or kinesthetic learner?

Here are some very brief summaries of the three learning styles:

 Visual learners want to see the information written down or watch someone else demonstrate what is required.

Auditory learners prefer to hear information and like to repeat things aloud when trying to remember something.

 Kinesthetic learners want to be physically involved in the learning experience and prefer "learning by doing."

These three preferences of receiving and presenting information are called *modalities of learning*.

Figure 1-3 shows the proportion of each learning style type in the general population. As you can see, most people prefer to learn when the information is presented visually.

Now sit back, grab a pencil, and answer the questions on the following learning-style assessment. It will help you to confirm your opinion of your learning preferences.

LEARNING-STYLE INVESTIGATION

In each case, choose the numbered item that is most like you. In some cases, none will be exactly like you. In other cases, several will be like you. Try to choose only one in each case.

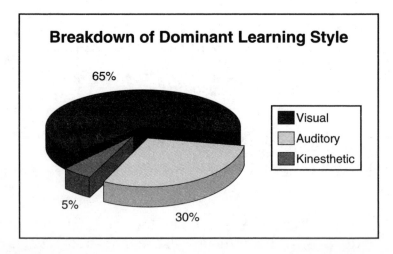

Breakdown of Dominant Learning Style

65%

Visual
Auditory
Kinesthetic

5%

30%

Figure 1-3

Case 1: I have an interest in learning to play golf. To explore this interest, I might find one of the following to be the most effective way to get started. It is most like me to

1. Talk to people who play golf to hear what they have to say
2. Take some lessons or hit a few balls at the driving range
3. Read books and magazines about it, get videos, and watch golf matches on TV

Case 2: A youngster wants me to learn how to use his computer to play games with him. To learn how to use the computer, I probably would select this as the first activity:

1. Read up on how to use a computer
2. Have someone tell me how to do it
3. Take a hands-on course at the public library, community college, or local computer store

Case 3: I am sitting with a child who is holding her favorite board game. She would like me to play with her. To learn the game, I would

1. Play the game and figure it out along the way
2. Have the child explain the rules to me
3. First, read the instructions to the game

Case 4: I have learned that there are wonderful ways to improve my mind. All of the following are good examples. The one I would choose to do first is

1. Read a new book
2. Participate in a discussion group
3. Learn a new craft

Case 5: To get exercise, I decide to take up walking. My ideal walk would be

1. On a treadmill so that I can watch TV or read while I walk

2. Walking with a radio to keep me company
3. Walking itself is so nice that I don't feel a need to do anything else

Case 6: The kinds of words I might use are

1. "Look at this." "See you later." "Oh, I see." "What a sight!"
2. "Here ... " "I get it." "Stay in touch." "What an upheaval!"
3. "Listen ... " "I didn't catch that." "I'll call you." "What a ruckus!"

Case 7: People point out that I

1. Doodle on my papers
2. Fidget in my seat or am always fooling with some object
3. Hum, mutter, or read aloud

Case 8: When I assemble a model airplane or another toy, I prefer to

1. Put the toy together, occasionally looking at the directions
2. Read the instructions out loud first, and then talk to myself during assembly
3. Read the instructions and look at the pictures, and then assemble it step by step

Case 9: To communicate with a friend, I would rather

1. Pick up the phone and have a conversation
2. Visit in person
3. Exchange letters or e-mail

Case 10: When I read a book,

1. I imagine myself as the hero or heroine. I create the scene in my mind in every detail used by the author

2. I notice the way the words flow and fit together like poetry

3. I like to get very comfortable first

Case 11: When I read a book,

1. Sometimes when I read a long sentence, I repeat it out loud to help me understand it

2. I like the way the book feels in my hands

3. I get lost in another world and lose track of time

Case 12: My idea of a good time is

1. Playing a rousing game of charades or other activities

2. Watching a great movie or reading a fine book

3. Going to a musical concert or singing with a group

Case 13: When someone is giving a speech

1. I am content to sit and listen

2. I look around the room to see what else is going on

3. I get agitated at having to sit still for a long time

This is the end of the assessment. In the next section, you will score yourself and be able to determine your dominant learning style.

LEARNING-STYLE INVESTIGATION RESULTS

You may have noticed that it was difficult to select just one of the choices. In some cases, you probably wanted to select two or more choices; in others, none matched your style at all. In the following cases, you will find a learning style that typically favors each of the choices you made. Count the number of auditory, visual, and kinesthetic choices you made. This will give you an indication of which learning style you prefer.

Case 1
1: Auditory
2: Kinesthetic
3: Visual

Case 2
1: Visual
2: Auditory
3: Kinesthetic

Case 3
1: Kinesthetic
2: Auditory
3: Visual

Case 4
1: Visual
2: Auditory
3: Kinesthetic

Case 5
1: Visual
2: Auditory
3: Kinesthetic

Case 6
1: Visual
2: Kinesthetic
3: Auditory

Case 7
1: Visual
2: Kinesthetic
3: Auditory

Case 8
1: Kinesthetic
2: Auditory
3: Visual

Case 9
1: Auditory
2: Kinesthetic, Visual,
   or Auditory
3: Visual

Case 10
1: Visual
2: Auditory
3: Kinesthetic

Case 11
1: Auditory
2: Kinesthetic
3: Visual

Case 12
1: Auditory, Kinesthetic,
   or Visual
2: Auditory or Visual
3: Auditory

Case 13
1: Auditory
2: Visual
3: Kinesthetic

So did the learning-style quiz confirm your previous opinion as to your learning preference, or did you learn something else about yourself? Your dominant style is the one for which you counted the highest score. The other two styles probably did not have a score of zero. So, there are some situations where you prefer to use the other two styles.

One of the authors typically tests as visual (when forced to select just one choice) but knows in her gut that she is strongly kinesthetic as well. She *has* to write things down to learn them, and if she does not do the driving cannot return to a location. Most people, in fact, rely on these three techniques to different degrees at different times. For example, to remember an errand that must be run, you may repeat it to yourself several times, while a trip to the hardware store for supplies may prompt you to write a list. You can train yourself to rely extensively on more than one modality to process information and create memories. The more you combine these modalities, the more efficient you will be at storing and recalling information.

USING LEARNING STYLES

To use your brain more fully, you need to use combinations of these methods to learn and recall pertinent information. Using a combination of visual and auditory methods creates more connections in the brain than using just one method. The more connections you use to store information, the more likely you will be able to recall it when required.

A friend of ours repeats to herself the thing she is trying to remember to do in an interesting rhyme or pattern (auditory), writes it down on a piece of paper and puts it next to her place mat where she will see it (visual and kinesthetic), and then tells her husband to remind her (auditory). The interesting thing is that she knows her husband will never remind her (he won't remember later), and he knows she doesn't really expect him to remind her (so he doesn't bother storing it). She never forgets anything! Are you surprised?

Why is it important in everyday life to be aware of learning preferences? We often think of learning as taking place in a formal environment such as a classroom or work. Nevertheless, we learn new information every day. Sometimes we are trying to learn and remember the errand we must run later in the day (and can forget afterward). Sometimes it is the new phone number of our best friend (which we do not want to forget).

Many times, we are not learning the information. We want someone else to remember something. If you notice the little signals indicating someone's dominant learning preference, you can present the information in the style that person needs.

The authors were part of a team conducting a national workshop for engineering professors. One of the things we taught them was to identify their learning style. One of the professors confessed that he was strongly kinesthetic. But what he thought so funny was that he now understood why his students would be so frustrated. They would come up to him after class, and no matter what the question was, he always tried to draw some sort of a picture to represent the question. They did not want a picture; they wanted him to clarify what he had said earlier. He needed to adjust his presentation style to match his students' learning style.

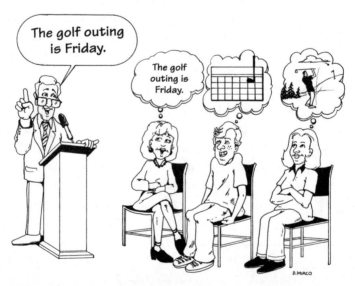

How auditory, visual, and kinesthetic learners think.

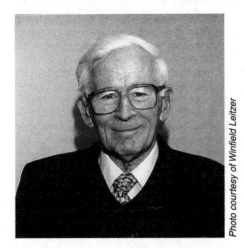

Photo courtesy of Winfield Leitzer

Older and Wiser

Glenn Austin, 77, learned about genealogy shortly before he retired as Director of Contracts for a division of Martin Marietta Corporation. Since then, to forward his avid interest, he has learned how to use vital records and census records (visual), paying attention to different spellings of the same-sounding name (auditory). He learned how to use the Family History Centers of the Mormon church; immigration, naturalization, military, and cemetery records; city directories; and many other information sources (visual) and search strategies (kinesthetic).

He learned how to use a computer (kinesthetic) for searching electronic bulletin board systems, e-mail, and the Web. He has met new people (auditory) and shared information through queries (visual), which are special requests made by genealogical researchers to each other.

Glenn finds the analysis of the data collected the most challenging element—a real-life detective activity.

Now he is able to apply his knowledge of computers to do new things, such as word processing (kinesthetic) to help keep minutes for his condominium board.

Glenn says, "Genealogy is the most fascinating thing I've ever done!" He is growing new brain connections at a rapid rate!

Now that you have an idea of what your dominant style is, there are two things for you to do. First, if you need to learn some new information in a quick and thorough manner, plan learning activities that maximize your dominant style.

- If you are a visual learner, feast your eyes with images and lots of text.

- If you prefer to learn in an auditory way, try books on tape or recite your lessons aloud. Use your voice and your ears to help you use this preferred style.

- A kinesthetic learner will want to devise activities where movement and touch are required. Make models, write notes, and use your hands to describe things to others and yourself.

Second, learn to develop your skills in the other two, less-dominant, learning styles. Life events often require you to use your nondominant style and still be effective at retaining information. You may be reading a magazine article, which supports a visual learner. You may be in an auditorium listening to someone speaking, which supports an auditory learner. You may be in a hands-on class, which supports a kinesthetic learner. It will be useful to you if you can benefit from all three styles.

Accommodate your personal preferences and begin to include others. If you have never been an avid reader, for example, find a subject you enjoy and start reading. The more techniques you use to store information, the more connections within your brain you'll create, and the more likely you will remember the information. (See Chapter 2, "The Intelligent Mind," for a more detailed explanation.) Exercise those brain cells! HUP, two, three, four. HUP, two, three, four . . .

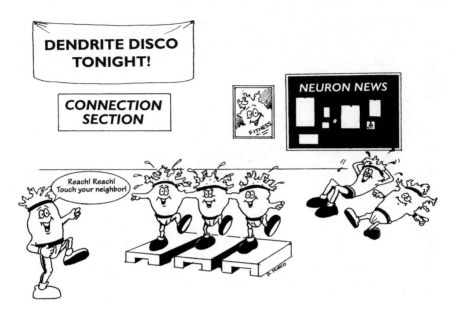

"No pain, no gain, no brain!"

One of the goals of the exercises in this book is to promote your development of all three modalities so that whatever situation arises, you will be able to maximize your acquisition and retention of information. In later chapters, you will have an opportunity to practice each of the three learning styles and increase your ease of use. In the meantime, fill in the following table with specific methods you can use to remember everyday examples of learning. Sometimes you need others to learn and remember something pertinent to your life, so we have included a few of those situations. Write as much as you can about how you will use these styles. We did the first one for you as an illustration. (Take a peek at that now.) You can use a combination of methods if you want, such as writing the item on a sticky note (kinesthetic) and sticking it where you will see it after work (visual reminder).

Learning Application	Visual	Auditory	Kinesthetic
Pick up bread after work.	Create a mental picture of picking up bread.	Repeat to yourself: put it into your *head* to pick up some *bread*.	Write it down three times on a piece of paper—*get bread*.
New phone number			
Lunch order for 10 visitors at work			
Friend's anniversary is next week.			
Car location in huge parking lot			
Your spouse needs to come home to meet the plumber.			
A friend is to pick you up at the airport.			

CONCLUSION

Using all of your learning-style possibilities exercises the various functional regions of your brain. You want to keep your seeing, listening, touching, smelling, and tasting skills fine-tuned and firing on all cylinders, like a well-tuned engine. In later chapters, you will have an opportunity to practice each of the three learning styles and increase your ease of use.

In this chapter, we emphasized your auditory, visual, and kinesthetic learning preferences. Remember the PET scans in Figure 1-2 that demonstrated the various areas targeted when processing information using the auditory, visual, and kinesthetic skills? In Chapter 2, you will discover that after the information passes into the brain, different areas are called upon to process the data.

REFERENCES:

1. Elizabeth Lasley, *Why on Earth Do We Sleep? (Brain-Work,* March/April 1998), 8.

The Intelligent Mind

Find Out How Your Brain Processes Information

KEY CONCEPTS

Brain Development
Multiple Intelligences
Memory and Its Acquisition
Multiple Intelligences Investigation

INTRODUCTION

Most of us are aware of how our body operates, ages, and repairs itself. We replace skin cells every day, for example, yet it takes approximately seven years before we have completed a full cycle and replaced all the old skin cells. It is also common knowledge that exercise benefits our overall health and can help us to resist the effects of aging on our bodies. Intimate knowledge of how our brain operates, ages, and repairs itself is not as common. Before you can take control of your mental processes, you must understand how the brain works.

In Chapter 1, "The Learning Styles of an Agile Mind,"you explored the concept of the visual, auditory, and kinesthetic learning preferences. While you were reading, whether or not you previously knew about the concept of learning styles, did you wonder why we have different learning preferences? Is one child born to be a visual learner, another an auditory learner, and still another a kinesthetic learner? Is this a preference we develop? Is it a preference we can influence or change?

To answer these questions, this chapter will tell you how the brain works. You will discover how your brain develops as you grow, and how different parts of your brain react while you are performing a variety of activities. You also will see how through disease, damage, or disuse, mental ability may be impaired or lost. This book is not intended to aid those who have lost mental ability due to disease or traumatic damage. However, it will show you how you can recover loss of mental ability as a result of disuse.

Many old notions about the brain and how we learn have been overturned during the past Decade of the Brain. It was commonly thought, for example, that we had only a fixed number of brain cells and that when we lost them to disease, trauma, or old age, we did not replace them in the way we renewed other body cells. We believed that brain cells could be destroyed but not replaced. We also anticipated that we would lose some of our mental agility as a normal result of the aging process. Brain research in this decade reversed those notions. Research just recently indicated that certain areas of the brain, such as the hippocampus, can generate replacement cells throughout your life span.[1] We also know now that we can grow new connections between the brain cells at a rapid rate *if we use our brains in new and novel ways, regardless of our age.*

In the same manner that understanding how an engine functions helps a mechanic to fine-tune a motor, understanding the functions of your brain will aid you in fine-tuning your mental abilities. Accordingly, some groundwork must be laid before delving directly into the many methods you can use to counteract the effects of aging on your mental processes.

GENERAL DEVELOPMENT OF THE BRAIN

Let's get started. Pictures of the brain are all around us in newspapers, magazines, and on television. Therefore, you probably already have a general idea of what the brain looks like. We're going to probe deeply into the structure of the brain so that you will know precisely why we want you to practice certain strategies and techniques and exactly what is happening as you reinforce your mental agility. Let's start with some of the vocabulary and imagery needed to talk about and visualize brain structure.

neuron—nerve cell in the brain

The neuron is the basis of the brain. It is estimated that the brain contains 100 billion neurons, which is roughly equivalent to the number of stars in the Milky Way galaxy.[2] Each neuron is a nerve cell composed of a center, named the *nucleus,* with long, slender axons and short, bristly dendrites.

axon—messenger of the brain
dendrite—message receiver in the brain

Neurons communicate with each other by passing nerve impulses down the axon of one neuron. At the end of each axon is a minute gap called the *synapse*

synapse—gap between axon and dendrites

As the nerve impulse reaches the end of the axon, a chemical, called a *neurotransmitter,* is released into the synapse. On the other side of the synapse is a dendrite of another cell that acts as the receiver for the signal.

neurotransmitter—a chemical released by the axon to
send and store messages across a synapse

In Figure 2-1, you can see the path the message follows from one neuron to another. This message travels from one

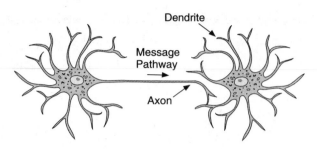

Figure 2-1 Connections between brain cells

neuron out its axon, is transmitted over the synapse, and travels up one of the dendrites of another neuron on its way to its destination. The message may be passed from neuron to neuron until it reaches the final destination. On the other hand, the neurotransmitters released into the synapse may alert multiple neurons at the same time. These message pathways are called *connections.*

connections—message pathways in the brain

Also present in the spaces between the neurons are trillions of *glial* cells, from the Greek word for *glue.* These cells support, sustain, and safeguard the neurons and may have a communications system of their own.

glial—glue-like cells that form a support for the neurons

The neurotransmitter performs a critical function in the creation of these communications connections. Each time a message is transmitted between cells, the chemical that is released into the synapse physically changes the receptor dendrite. Bristly spikes build on the dendrite as a result of the interaction of the chemical neurotransmitter and the dendrite. It is the repetition of this chemical reaction along the message route that strengthens the connection. You will learn in Chapter 4, "Develop a Brawny Brain," how to use rehearsal to make a memory stronger. (Visit the Web site www.mentalagility.com to view an animation of this phenomenon.)

The basis for these communications connections already can be identified approximately 10 weeks after conception when the brain is merely one-half inch long.[3] Neurons begin pushing their way from the neural tube deep within the interior of the fetus's brain to the outside margins, with newer neurons pushing past older neurons. Neurons travel along glial fibers much like traveling down a highway toward their final destination with the assistance of proteins and chemical cues.[4] By five months into the pregnancy, the fetus's brain is now two inches long, and the migration of neurons to the outer layers of the brain is almost complete.[5]

Early Brain Development

During development, a baby's brain is a maze of neurons much different in structure from the adult's brain. One interesting example is vision development. To develop vision, nerve fibers from the retina must grow to extend far enough through the brain to reach the visual thalamus (see Figure 2-2), and from there, axons reach to the outer layers of the cortex, before the cortex even exists.

cortex—the folded outer layer of the brain

A study by Carla J. Shatz,[6] professor of neurobiology at Stanford University, demonstrated the existence of transient support "scaffolding" in the developing brain that aids in developing vision but disappears after the brain's growth is finished. Special types of neurons, *subplate neurons,* suddenly appear just below the final destination at the visual cortex and function to bolster and direct the axons to their proper location. Then these subplate neurons disappear. These and other neurons that act as temporary support structures, along with the proteins and chemical cues previously mentioned, prevent the axons from wandering into incorrect areas and impairing brain functions. Some disabilities, such as cerebral palsy, autism, epilepsy, schizophrenia, and dyslexia are thought to be a result of wandering axons or improper connections.[7]

LEFT VISUAL FIELD   **RIGHT VISUAL FIELD**

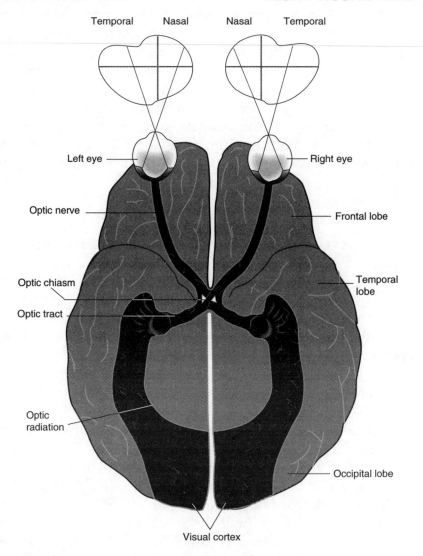

Figure 2-2 Pathway from retina to visual cortex

At birth, the brain weighs approximately three-quarters of a pound. The migrating axons have reached the correct general area but not necessarily the exact site. The neurons in the visual cortex alone form about 2,500 connections per neuron at birth, and with proper stimulation, this rapidly increases to 18,000 connections per neuron after about six months. Stimulation, including touching, speaking to the baby, and presenting different images, helps the brain increase efficiency and select correct sites. Research demonstrates that babies who are not stimulated have brains 20 percent to 30 percent smaller than normal.[8] This process of stimulation and mental reaction is much like fine-tuning a station on the old-style radio dial: If the message gets close to the proper site, but not exactly where it needs to be, the result is not as clear as if the tuning were exact. Each time the message is sent, the tuning becomes more effective, until at last, with sufficient testing of the connections, the signal is processed clear and free of static.

From birth, the baby learns to be efficient at transferring auditory, visual, and/or kinesthetic information. As you read to a child and point out the words, you are stimulating the auditory and visual aspects of learning. Taking a child's hand and tracing the letters reinforces the kinesthetic qualities. It is important that the child is exposed repeatedly to all the learning preferences in order to fine-tune the circuits used for each technique (more on that in just a bit). The more techniques the child can call upon during the school years, the more likely the child will be considered a success in the traditional school setting. The traditional school setting primarily supports visual and auditory learners.

As the brain learns what the correct representations are and which paths are most efficient at transmitting this information, it keeps the most-effective pathways and prunes the less-efficient ones. Connections, which are used on a regular basis and thus become fine-tuned, are retained, while other connections, which are inefficient or not used at all, are eliminated.[9] As many as 600 connections may be eliminated *per second* during this pruning period. After the synapses and axons are operating correctly, the efficiency of the mental processing is dependent on genetic, environmental (including nutritional and sociological), psychological, and educational factors.[10]

The time after birth is extremely critical. For the first couple of years, the child's brain is most malleable. After approximately 8 to 10 years of age, the brain is not as adaptable to change. That is why young children who suffer brain injuries recover more quickly and completely than adults with the same brain injuries. We begin to develop our learning preferences before we reach school age. We already know whether we like to learn and how we want to go about it before we ever reach kindergarten. This is why the quality of the interactions of the parents or caregivers with the child are extremely critical to the learning process and the future success of the student. If you have been successful in learning in formal school settings, you probably are successful in real-life settings such as your job. If you have been unsuccessful in learning in the past, or if you are experiencing difficulty holding on to information from day to day, you can improve your capabilities. You can literally "change your mind" and be more efficient and reliable. But assuming you are an adult, you need to know the facts about how your brain operates in order to affect the processes. Please keep reading . . .

The Adult Brain

By the time the baby becomes an adult, the brain weighs approximately three pounds. This increase in weight is due to the increase in neuron size and the tremendous increase in the number of connections formed among the neurons since birth. Imagine trying to take billions of neurons formed in layers and trying to fit them into the skull. It is similar to trying to fit a piece of newspaper into a small box. Crumpling it in on itself would be a good solution. The layers of neurons form the gray matter and enfold the trillions of axons passing through the brain and interconnecting the neurons. The myelin sheaths covering the axons are white; this region therefore is described as *white matter.*[11] The cortex makes up 80 percent of the brain's volume and is the convoluted mass normally imagined when the word "brain" is mentioned.

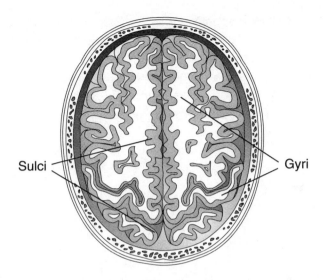

Sulci

Gyri

Figure 2-3 Top view of the brain showing both hemispheres

The grooves and folds, named *sulci* and *gyri*, respectively, that appear on the surface of the cortex are used as landmarks or reference points to locations within the brain (see Figure 2-3).

> **sulci**—*grooves in the cortex*
> **gyri**—*folds in the cortex*

One of the deepest of the sulci divides the cortex from the front to the back into two hemispheres. The two hemispheres are connected primarily by a thick bundle of nerves named the *corpus callosum*, (See Figure 2-4).

Just as bodies have the same general configuration (the head bone's connected to the neck bone, the neck bone's connected to the shoulder bone . . .), everybody's brain has the same anatomical parts. Each of us has two hemispheres, a corpus callosum, grooves, and folds. These grooves (sulci) and folds (gyri) are so standardized in location that they are used as landmarks or reference points to locations and activities within the brain.

Left Hemisphere   Right Hemisphere

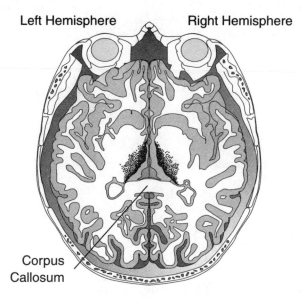

Corpus
Callosum

Figure 2-4 The hemispheres and their bridge, the corpus callosum

Brain Function Location

Some functions carried out by the brain have been identified as to location. The more basic functions of life, such as breathing, are located close to the base and the spinal column in the brainstem. The cortex handles the higher-reasoning skills, such as language, math, and musical abilities; and the appreciation of humor.

The Hemispheres

Common phrases overheard these days are *right-brained* and *left-brained.* These phrases refer to the primary location for specific mental activities within the brain structure (see Figure 2-5). The left hemisphere communicates with and controls the right side of the body, while the right hemisphere communicates with and controls the left side of the body. Although both hemispheres communicate with each other and share some functions, one hemisphere is considered dominant. The dominant hemisphere is the site for thought processes more involved in detailed and sequential analysis.

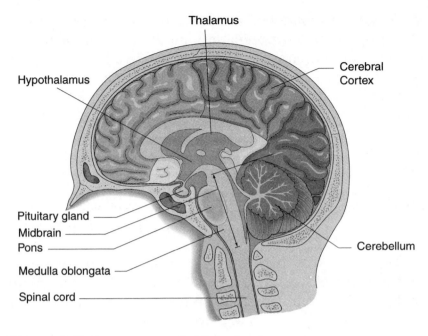

Figure 2-5 Basic structure of the brain

Whichever hemisphere is dominant, it is the other hemisphere that holds appreciation of forms and humor, mental arousal, physiological readiness to respond, orientation in space, recognition of voice timbre, musical talent, and appreciation of things that do not lend themselves to verbal descriptions.[12] This hemisphere is considered to be the home site for global thought processes that can be described as the "Aha!" response, which is exhibited when a sudden understanding of a concept occurs without the ability to describe how the understanding was achieved. It often is assumed that the left hemisphere controls the verbal and analytical processes, while the right hemisphere handles the artistic, emotional, abstract relationships. This is true for only a portion of the population.

There are some clues, however, as to which hemisphere is dominant. Approximately 99 percent of the right-handed population and 56 percent of the left-handed population write with the hand in a noninverted position. One percent of the right-handed population and 44 percent of the left-handed population write with the hand in an inverted position (see Figure 2-6). Dr. Jerre Levy performed experiments that revealed that the inverted hand position is a biological marker indicating that the hemisphere considered dominant for analytical specialization is on the same side as the writing hand. For those people who write with the hand in a noninverted position, the hemisphere opposite that hand is dominant. For discussion purposes, and because it is the case for most of the population, we will consider the left hemisphere of the brain to be the site for verbal and analytical abilities for the rest of this text.

We have all heard jokes regarding the differences between men and women. There is a biological basis for many of the qualities men and women find confusing about each other. For example, men and women differ at a very basic level from the description just given for the dominant hemisphere. While men's verbal abilities are predominantly

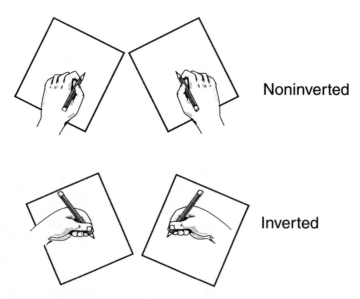

Figure 2-6 Hand position as a marker for hemisphere dominance

stored in a centralized location in the left hemisphere, a woman's verbal abilities are more diffusely located on both sides of the brain. This might explain why men have a slightly more difficult time expressing their emotions. They have to get the emotional information from the right hemisphere across the primary bridge (corpus callosum) to their verbal abilities in the left hemisphere, whereas women have some verbal abilities already located on the same side as their emotions.[13] See Chapter 3, "Teach Your Brain Agility," for more details of gender differences.

Each hemisphere is further divided into lobes.

Each lobe has generalized functions. The *frontal* lobes have the capability to plan for the future, control movement, integrate emotional responses, and produce speech. The *parietal* lobes receive and process information received from the senses—such as pain, taste, and smell—and are involved with logic and mathematical processes. The *occipital* lobes handle vision. The *temporal* lobes hear and interpret language, tones, sound patterns, and music; and participate in emotion. The *limbic* lobe is responsible for sexual, emotional, and memory processing[14] (see Figure 2-7).

Researchers at the University of Toronto's Baycrest Center for Geriatric Care announced that the frontal lobes are where humor is processed. People with a brain injury to a frontal lobe don't get punch lines. They prefer slapstick

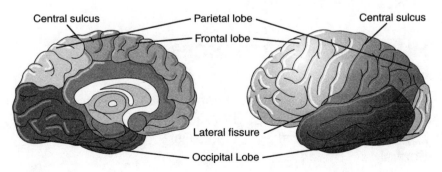

Figure 2-7 Side and central cross sectional views of the lobes

humor! The people with damage to that area had difficulty selecting the correct response to a joke similar to this one:

A teenager is being interviewed for a summer job.

"You'll get $50 a week to start off," says his boss. "Then after a month, you'll get a raise to $75 a week."

Punch-line selection:

A. "I'd like to take the job. When can I start?" (straightforward logical choice)

B. "That's great! I'll come back in a month." (correct funny choice—original punch line)

C. "Hey boss, your nose is too big for your face!" (slapstick ending—right-frontal damaged patients are likely to choose this one)[15]

Now that we have led you through a discussion of the brain's general anatomy and structure, let's talk about the brain, learning, and intelligences so that we can apply this information to our learning capability. You know your abilities and talents. Maybe you are talented at fixing things, cooking, writing, solving crossword puzzles, cheering other people up, or gardening. Before you begin reading about intelligences (and all these "talents" are actually forms of intelligence), review your skills and abilities. Then see whether you recognize yourself in any of these intelligences. The following facts and figures will provide you with some interesting information if you have ever dealt with someone who has had a stroke or other brain injury.

MULTIPLE INTELLIGENCES

Seven Intelligences

Linguistic	Bodily-Kinesthetic
Musical	Personal
Logical-Mathematical	Naturalist
Spatial	

As a framework for our discussion of more specific capabilities of the brain, we will use Howard Gardner's theory of multiple intelligences.[16] Gardner feels that too much importance has been placed on the types of skills and talents required to score well on standardized intelligence tests. A person who scores a high *intelligence quotient* (IQ) does so as the result of performing well on certain linguistic, spatial, and mathematical tasks. Gardner holds that there are at least seven intelligences that should be valued equally: linguistic, musical, logical-mathematical, spatial, bodily-kinesthetic, naturalist, and personal (which includes interpersonal and intrapersonal).

We will designate general sites for each of these mental activities within the brain. Remember that we are choosing the left hemisphere as the dominant hemisphere. If you are right-hemisphere dominant, you should switch the designated locations shown here to the other side of the brain. Also, when we discuss an activity (for example, mathematics), we will point out the area in which research shows the activity is concentrated. However, when you actually "do math" in a practical application, other areas of the brain, such as language and spatial abilities, usually are involved. One area is not independent of the others.

Linguistic Intelligence

 "The Father of Waters rolls unvexed to the sea" was General Grant's telegraph to President Lincoln on the fall of Vicksburg during the Civil War. What a melodic, stunning report. Someone not so facile with the language might have said, "Enemy defeated at Vicksburg. Mississippi River now under Union control." Lincoln, himself, days later while delivering the Gettysburg Address, used the robust passage "Four score and seven years ago" to replace the austere phrase "In 1776."

Some people, such as Grant and Lincoln, possess such a high linguistic intelligence that their ability to create finely crafted sentences progresses beyond precision and accuracy into the realm of an art form. Whereas the left hemisphere specializes in understanding literal meaning, there is good evidence that the right hemisphere helps in understanding and generating metaphors, humor, and irony. Subjects with damage to the right hemisphere understand words in an extremely literal manner. When asked to show appreciation for a performance and "give someone a hand," they would try to find a toy hand to give. When asked to complete jokes, the result would be senseless, awkward, and not in the least humorous.[17] The creative ability and imaginative use of words, located largely in the right hemisphere, is the essence that raises technical merit to a creative painting of pictures that evoke strong emotions and vivid interactions.

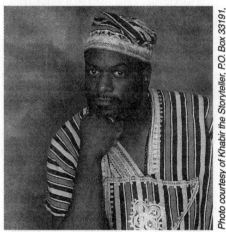

Photo courtesy of Khabir the Storyteller, P.O. Box 33191, Indianapolis, IN 46203

Khabir the Storyteller relates African and African-American stories and folktales in the oral tradition. Khabir may spin traditional African folktales in the style of the griot, he may use first-person interpretation in the character of Martin Delany (an African-American Civil War officer), or he may use some other character. In any case, audience participation is an essential part of Khabir's presentations. Khabir, at 50 years old, has been a professional storyteller for 10 years.

"I like sharing stories that enhance understanding of African and African-American history and culture and reinforce good social values," Khabir says.

He likes to use stories that are stimulating, sometimes humorous, and presented in an entertaining way.

According to Gardner in *Frames of Mind,* everyone can aspire to master four main objectives:

1. *Rhetoric*—use of language to convince another individual that your opinion is correct

2. *Mnemonic*—use of language to remember other information

3. *Explanation*—use of language for teaching and learning

4. *Metalinguistic*—use of language for analyzing previous statements for clarification or correction

Mastery of language and its uses requires expert knowledge and use of phonology (word sounds that interact), semantics (the meaning of words), and syntax (rules of word order to use as expected or changed to draw attention to a particular idea or image). Individual elements of a task (in this case, phonology, semantics, and syntax) may be localized within a specific area of the brain. These elements and their respective areas are activated in any number of combinations to complete that task.

The specific areas designated for these three elements are shown in the figure. These areas are referred to as Broca's area (linguistic production) and Wernicke's area (comprehension of linguistics). The area for processing sign language is located just below Wernicke's area[18] (see Figure 2-8).

These areas are not the only ones used for linguistics. Marble-sized areas of neurons, primarily scattered through the left temporal and parietal lobes, specialize in functions such as nouns, individual rules of grammar, and production of verbs. You might be interested to know what parts of the brain exhibit the most activity when thinking and speaking words.

 Musical Intelligence

Interest in music may be expressed in different forms: listening to music, performing music, and composing music. While some people just "muddle through," composers are

described as constantly hearing in their minds the notes and tones of their lives. It is not an act of will but rather a way of life, much like breathing or walking for those of us not so blessed.

Many children generate spontaneous songs in their early years, but by the age of six or seven, this ceases for the majority. Children then seem to rely primarily on the standardized tunes they are taught. Only a few continue to create music.

Most of the information available on music generation comes from observing musicians who have experienced physical trauma to the brain as a result of stroke or other brain damage. Damage to the left hemisphere exhibits *aphasia* (verbal-production impairment) or *amusia* (musical-production impairment). Subjects could talk coherently and not be able to function musically (amusia) or not be able to verbalize (aphasia) and still perform or compose. Some people documented in literature have had strokes that affected the left side of their brain, leaving them unable to speak a single word; yet they could sing song after song. Sometimes they required a trigger mechanism, depending on the damage, such as another person starting the song or a record to give them a "jog."

Although Dr. Wetzel's grandmother was not a documented case, her experience is germane. She could not respond verbally to any question but could sing her gospel hymns for hours. However, she needed to hear a recording to get her started. In addition, Alzheimer's patients are often able to sing or play an instrument long after their recognition of friends and families has passed.

Although one of the main areas that facilitates music production also assists in verbal skills, music seems to be of the form of a symbolic or graphic system as opposed to an alphabetic, semantic system and thus is related closely to mathematical skills.

PET scanning was used in a study performed on 10 right-handed performers, each with at least 15 years of experience and self-rated as good to excellent sight readers. The study included two categories common to all instruments: sight reading and playing the instrument.[19] For this study, the in-

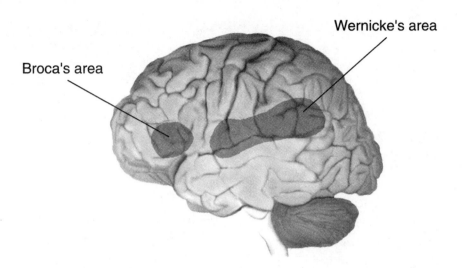

Wernicke's area

Broca's area

Figure 2-8 Location of Broca's area and Wernicke's area.

strument was a keyboard. Reading a musical score without playing operates both hemispheres' visual centers, as expected. Instead of stimulating the linguistic centers, the left occipitoparietal junction, normally used when processing spatial information, is activated. This agrees with the manner in which musicians use distance between notes on the staff to locate the next pitch and supports the theory that spatial abilities are fundamental to musical intelligence. As a matter of fact, the distance from the area of the brain activated when listening to low C to that area activated when listening to middle C is the same distance as that from the area listening to middle C to that listening to high C.[20]

The drawing in Figure 2-9 indicates the areas activated when listening to scales. Notice that listening to a musical composition (as opposed to the predictability of scales) activated the same cortical areas and an additional arc in the right hemisphere. Listening to music (scales being classified as practice, not music) affects the emotional and imaginative areas of the right hemisphere, whereas scales do not.

You can see the areas fundamental to playing music. Music requires fine motor control, and the picture shows the

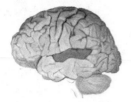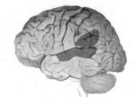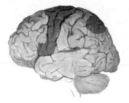

Figure 2-9 Left: Listening to scales. Center: Listening to musical scores. Right: Playing music

primary motor and premotor areas active. Although music processing is located in both hemispheres, the more experienced a musician becomes in processing musical tones, the more the process seems to be located in the left hemisphere.[21] As skills become activated automatically, as opposed to having to concentrate on how to perform the action, they are considered rote performances and become located in a separate area of the brain in the left hemisphere.

The area of the brain thought to lift the technically correct performer to the level of an artist is the right hemisphere. Many people can play adequately, but this does not indicate a creative instinct. Those composers and performers who hear their lives as musical interludes have a depth of activation in the right hemisphere that may at various times seem a blessing or a burden.

 Logical-Mathematical Intelligence

A pure mathematician deals not so much with numbers, as we remember our arithmetic classes, but with extreme abstractions that are built with reasoning and many lines of proofs into even more abstract results. To many people, these abstractions often seem to have no reference to the "real" world. It may be difficult for many people who have had bad experiences in the past, to think of mathematics as a potential art form. However, as is the case with the other intelligences discussed so far, the creative genius that sparks new theories and applications seems to reside in the right hemisphere. (A lot of readers would simply like to know where the *average* mathematical skills are based!)

The only available information regarding the location of mathematical abilities is from observation of those individuals who have suffered damage to the brain through an accident or stroke, or who required surgery. *Gerstmann Syndrome* is the designation for damage to the left parietal lobes and the temporal and occipital association areas adjoining them (part of the angular gyrus). Damage to these areas reduces the ability to orient oneself in space, understand certain grammatical structures (such as prepositional phrases and passive constructions), tell left from right, and perform numerical calculations. It also creates difficulty in drawing. The syndrome is characterized by damaging effects to the association cortexes in the posterior areas of the dominant hemisphere—those associated with recognizing ordered arrays and patterns visually (see Figure 2-10).

Deficits in calculation abilities can be grouped into three main categories:

1. *Alexic and agraphic acalculia*—difficulty in reading and writing numbers

2. *Spatial acalculia*—difficulty in dealing with the spatial organization of written numbers

3. *Anarithmetria*—difficulty with the calculation itself

The first two types of deficits (difficulty in visualizing numbers) are linked to the visual system and/or associative memory areas. Damage to the posterior portion of the left hemisphere, near Wernicke's area, results in the calculation disability.

Essential to the logical-mathematical ability, the frontal lobes play an important part in organization skills. The ability to plan a strategy to achieve a specific goal is housed in this area. Damage to the frontal lobes leaves an individual with not only an inability to plan a problem-solving strategy but also the inability to set goals and follow through in everyday life.

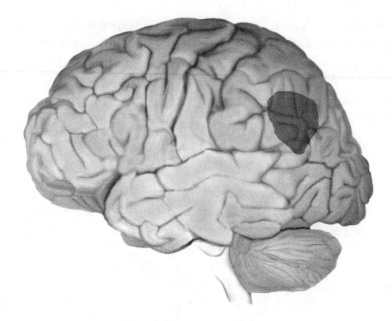

Figure 2-10 Area for mathematical calculation

The ability to handle mathematics successfully is somewhat dependent on the strength of the individual's spatial abilities (as in music). Also of importance is the ability to understand fully numerical relationships and concepts. Because this requires a sense of intuition and feeling instead of sequential proof, this ability is lodged in the right hemisphere. Again, this is rather similar to the organization of the brain when dealing with music. Music seems to lend a sense of order and beauty to expressions that mathematicians and scientists enjoy and appreciate. Teaching young children a musical instrument or exposing them to music, especially the classics, helps to organize their thought pro-cesses and make children more successful in mathematics.[22]

 Spatial Intelligence

Second only to research on the linguistic operations of the brain is research regarding spatial abilities. Perhaps so much research is available on spatial abilities because it is something, like language, that we are all called upon to use. In addition, this is one of the primary mental abilities often tested on IQ tests.

An example of spatial abilities is the capability to answer the question, "Is the top of a horse's tail located above or below the level of its chin?" To answer the question, you must visualize
the horse's formation. Spatial skills consist of abilities to

1. Experience the world in three dimensions.

2. Understand scale models and recognize objects in unusual orientations.

3. Recall visual images in rich detail.[23]

The posterior (rear) portions of the right hemisphere are more crucial for spatial reasoning, although damage to the left hemisphere can cause a slight decrease in this ability. For most individuals, the right hemisphere is dominant (see Figure 2-11).

In general, men perform better at spatial tasks, especially rotation of objects, mathematical reasoning, and navigating through a route. Studies have been performed using men and women with normal hormonal levels and women who were exposed to prenatal and neonatal doses of the hormone androgen (due to genetic defects or the pregnant mother taking steroids). The increased spatial abilities apply to the women exposed to androgens early in development. Women who had not been exposed to the hormone did not perform as well. However, they did perform better at matching items, arithmetic calculation, recalling landmarks on a route, and precision tasks. They also showed greater verbal fluency.

Because the hormone testosterone is present in both men and women (at different levels), the next question raised is whether a direct relationship exists between the level of testosterone and spatial ability. Is there an optimum level of the hormone for increased spatial abilities? There is a range on the high end for women's normal levels and the low end

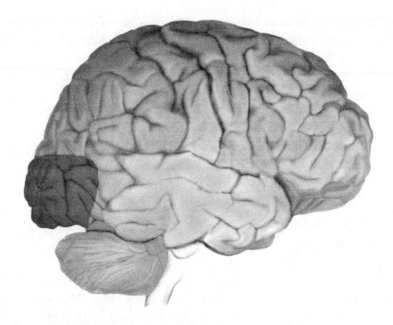

Figure 2-11 Location of spatial ability in both hemispheres (right dominant)

for men's normal levels that is optimum. Too high on the men's scale or too low on the women's scale reduces the spatial abilities. An individual's spatial abilities also fluctuate during the normal hormonal cycles for women and men (testosterone levels for men are lower in the spring than in the fall).[24]

Bodily-Kinesthetic Intelligence

Not often regarded as an intelligence, body intelligence is the ability to use the body in highly differentiated and skilled ways and the ability to use other objects skillfully.[25] Examples include acting, the skilled movements of the hands and fingers of an instrumentalist, ballet, and gymnastics. Figure 2-12 shows the primary areas for motor skills and control.

The *Supplementary Motor Area* (SMA) predetermines the general path of a movement or series of movements. Even as simple a task as waving good-bye can become impossible to perform and impossible to learn if the SMA is damaged.[26] The premotor cortex and the basal ganglia aid in the planning and implementation of the path of the movement. The posterior parietal lobe, important in spatial ability, interacts with the premotor cortex.

The process of movement actually is accomplished with two loops through the system: a complex loop and a motor loop. The complex loop begins with instructions from the frontal lobes. The instructions then are fed through the basal ganglia and caudate nucleus portions and are sent to the thalamus. Then the information is fed back through the frontal lobes and into the motor loop. The motor loop begins with M1, where fine motor control is located. Some of the neurons located in M1 have direct access to the spinal column. The cerebellum is included in the pathway, because it appears to be the site of automatic motor responses (those skills that are "second nature").

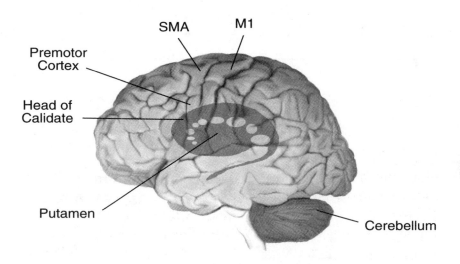

Figure 2-12 Location of the motor control system

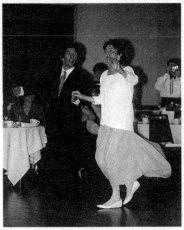

Photo courtesy of Amy Aldrich

Automatic Motor Response

Ball Room Dancing is an example of automatic motor response *(AMR). Sharon Mulgrew and Bryan Umeki have practiced their dancing so often that they now are operating from
AMR. At the beginning, they had to concentrate deeply to learn
the movements. It is this AMR feature of their brains that allows
them to finally enjoy dancing.*

While learning to drive, one of the authors' sisters com-
plained that is was hard to work the manual transmission.
Her dad quipped that it would be hard at the beginning, but
after a while, it would become automatic.

Some activities are performed so often that they become
automatic motor responses (such as actions performed by a
skilled typist or pianist). The reactions are too quick for true
interaction between the stimulus (typing an "a") and the
reasoning abilities (Where is the letter "a" on a keyboard?
There it is. Hit it.). When children first begin to write, the
shapes and drawing mechanisms for each letter are matters
of intense concentration. After years of practice, writing becomes automatic. The movements are stored in memory as

a single associate memory, ready to access and process in a fraction of a second. These memory associations, thought to be stored in the cerebellum, are like computer routines. The instructions are carried out in a specific order at an extremely rapid pace.

Sometimes skills become so automatic that it is difficult to explain the details to someone else. And slowing down the actions to explain the details often causes an error in the process. This explains why most people have difficulty writing with their opposite hand. The instructions in your brain are for the directions and movements of the dominant hand, and at times, you would have to move in a different manner for the other hand.[27]

Personal Intelligence

Personal intelligence is one of the less distinct and comparable intelligences. Personal intelligence consists of intrapersonal and interpersonal knowledge. *Intrapersonal* knowledge is knowledge of self—an ability to draw upon, evaluate, and symbolize your own feelings. Examples of intrapersonal experts might be a novelist or a wise elder. *Interpersonal* knowledge incorporates knowledge of relationships among people; the ability to notice details of others' feelings, facial expressions, and tone; and the ability to influence others. Examples of interpersonal experts are politicians, teachers, and counselors.

The frontal lobes are the meeting place between the information from the posterior regions (involved in processing sensory information, including perceptions of others) and the limbic system (involved in motivational and emotional functions). Frontal lobes are where the self meets the outside world and the knowledge of self appears to reside. Noticing body language is a major component of interpersonal knowledge. The ability to notice fine details of the face and expressions is activated in the posterior region of the right hemisphere. This is the same area used to process spatial abilities. (Spatial abilities seem to be important for most of the intelligences.)

The intimate knowledge and understanding of your inner self, combined with foresight and insight, are essential to interpersonal and intrapersonal expertise. Your emotional behavior and personality, in combination with expert evaluative skills (judgment) also are critical to your relationships with others. Figure 2-13 indicates the areas of the brain that regulate these skills.

Self-knowledge can be misleading. Take young children, for example. At the age of 6 or 7, children become concerned with the acquisition of skills and knowledge. Peer pressure and the need to please oneself and one's parents become quite influential. Influence by others that can be destructive at times may include adults and other children dissuading a young girl or boy from an interest in a nontraditional role. The child begins to doubt his or her own interests and abilities and chooses a secondary, more acceptable goal. The personal intelligence might be the one most important for each person's satisfaction with life.

Naturalist Intelligence

Lately Gardner has been considering other forms of intelligences. The newest is that of naturalist intelligence. Not much has been written about this while Dr. Gardner refines his concepts. However, this much is clear: People who possess naturalist intelligence are attuned with nature. We sus-

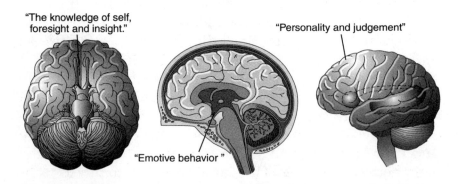

Figure 2-13

pect that they know the names of plants and animals. If they have auditory skills, they likely know birds by their calls. Weather is not a mystery to them. They are always aware of their surroundings and love to spend time outdoors. Their houseplants thrive, and their gardens are stunning. We look forward to learning more about the naturalist as Dr. Gardner's work progresses.

MEMORY

How do we acquire memories? The memory-formation system is made up of the hippocampus, the limbic thalamus, and the basal forebrain. Information is obtained through the senses, passed through the memory-formation system, and transferred to permanent storage in the outer layers of the cortex (see Figure 2-14). For information that you need on a temporary basis, nerve cells adjust existing proteins to hold the memory until you no longer need it. Then when the need is over, the neurons return to their original state, and you forget. If the information is something you want to store permanently, entirely new types of proteins are manufactured, new genes are "switched on," and permanent changes to the connections in the structure of the brain are created.[28] So there is a difference in the brain's activation for a temporary piece of information, such as what you need to buy at the store, and a more permanent memory, such as your new telephone number.

Recent evidence indicates that the transfer of the information from the hippocampus to the cortex for permanent storage occurs while we sleep. For the maximum efficiency of memory transfer, you need to have deep sleep within the first two hours of sleep and *rapid eye movement* (REM) sleep later in the night, preferably toward the end of the sleep cycle. The same neurons activated earlier in the day, when the information first was introduced, fire in the same pattern and appear to download the information through the neuron connections to the cortex.

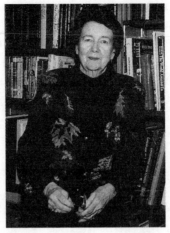

Photo courtesy of Winfield Leitzer

Older and Wiser

Rosemary Austin, 77, possesses naturalist intelligence. The Weather Channel is one of her favorites. She is very interested in and conscious of the times for sunrise and sunset, ocean tides, moon phases, and the like. Her many and varied houseplants qualify her for a "green thumb" award. She never gets lost and always knows the shortest route to any destination.

She also possesses linguistic intelligence. Since retiring from a successful teaching career, she has written several novels and is very active in several romance writer associations.

No matter what our age, we can create new connections within the brain. It is repeated exposure to new information that grows these connections. The more connections we have, the deeper the brain's resources upon which to call. As adults, we can produce and fine-tune neuron connections much as a baby creates new connections after birth. We also can grow new cells, particularly in the hippocampus (the area helping us to store new memories and continue learning). Research such as the Seattle Longitudinal and Baltimore Longitudinal studies prove that not only can you maintain mental agility and performance as you age into your 80s and beyond, you

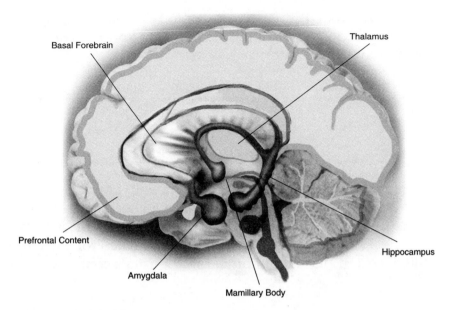

Figure 2-14 Memory storage systems

can regain performance levels you may have had in the past (see Chapters 6, "Regain an Agile Brain," and 7, "Enjoy Your Ageless Mental Agility," for more details).

Areas of processing that are used frequently increase in size and move into some of the surrounding areas previously allocated for other functions. If you don't use it, you do indeed lose it!

MULTIPLE INTELLIGENCES INVESTIGATION

Recall that Howard Gardner believes that there are at least seven intelligences that should be valued equally: linguistic, musical, logical-mathematical, spatial, bodily-kinesthetic, naturalist, and personal. Knowing your strengths will provide valuable information to you. First you will know what types of learning will come easily to you. Second, you will be able to understand, and learn to compensate for, the types of learning that are difficult for you.

Take a moment to speculate as to what your strengths might be. Choose three of the intelligences you feel you possess. Write them in the spaces below.

1. _____

2. _____

3. _____

The following sets of questions will help you to identify your own intelligence strengths. Place a check next to each sentence that describes you. Count the number of options you checked for each set of characteristics listed for each intelligence and place that number in the Totals column.

Intelligence	Indicators	Totals
Naturalist	____ You notice patterns in nature.	
	____ You know what the weather is supposed to be like.	
	____ You know the names of many animals and plants.	
	____ You recognize and classify minerals.	
	____ You know what the phase of the moon is.	
		Total: _____
Bodily-Kinesthetic	____ You enjoy activities where you can move about.	
	____ You seldom injure yourself while exercising.	
	____ You learn dance steps quickly.	
	____ You would rather make something than read about it.	
	____ You love to play sports rather than watch others play.	
		Total: _____

Logical-Mathematical

___ Puzzles and games are very easy for you to master.
___ Doing math is fun for you.
___ You are fascinated by machines.
___ You like to solve mysteries.
___ You tend to win arguments often.

Total: _____

Spatial

___ You seldom get lost.
___ You like to design new arrangements of furniture.
___ You can imagine what something will look like after it is built.
___ You like to do jigsaw puzzles.
___ You know whether or not a glass will overflow if you empty the rest of the milk bottle into it.

Total: _____

Linguistic

___ You love words.
___ Poetry is like music to you.
___ You have a large vocabulary.
___ You have written short stories, poetry or a novel.
___ You speak, read or understand several languages.

Total: _____

Musical

___ You sing, hum or whistle often.
___ You remember tunes easily.
___ You hear rhythm in everyday sound.
___ You play one or more instruments.
___ You have composed music.

Total: _____

Intrapersonal

___ You understand who you are.
___ You know your strengths.
___ You know your weaknesses.
___ You know what you want.
___ You are in control of your emotions most of the time.

Total: _____

Interpersonal	___You understand other people very well.
☺	___You often become the leader in any group you join.
	___Other people tend to come to you for advice.
	___You want to improve the human condition.
	___You work well in a group.
	Total: ___

Gardner thinks that we may have several intelligences and that we have all of them to one extent or another. If your totals are three or more, that indicates a strength in that intelligence.

With regard to Gardner's multiple intelligences, maximize your use of your dominant intelligences. Yet take the opportunity to develop those that are not your native intelligences. Intelligence is to a great extent learned. Experts still debate the "nature versus nurture" character of intelligence. While they debate, read on and see how much you can impact the quality of your intelligences.

We want you to be more aware of the activities of your marvelously designed brain. Often we don't appreciate being able to do something until we no longer can do it well or not at all. Picture how you felt when you couldn't breathe easily the last time you had a stuffy nose.

However, we want you to notice how you go about learning and what subject areas (intelligences) you prefer to learn, so that you can appreciate your mind, right now, and begin to exercise the various abilities of your brain.

The discussions regarding the various types of intelligences show that different parts of the brain are used for different functioning requirements. Some areas of your brain are stronger than others due to use. Remember as you use specific areas of your brain and they receive stimulation from the outside world, axons and dendrites in those areas are created and enlarged. But notice that if you exercise one of your skills, you still may be weak in other areas. That makes sense. If you are bench pressing weights to strengthen your arms and back, you will not be strengthening your legs. You need to exercise all areas of your body and so you also

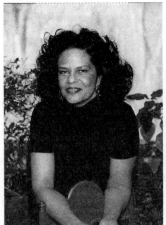

Photo courtesy of Winfield Leitzer

Older and Wiser

After raising three children and working 16 years as a dry cleaner, Doris Waller, 53, looked for a change of pace. She had always enjoyed housekeeping, so she took on a job with a maid service. After a highly successful first year, Doris struck out on her own. Now she is president of her own housekeeping service, D&W Cleaning, Inc., which serves professional offices and private homes. Doris has kept busy learning entrepreneurial skills for her expanding business. Her current task is mastering the computer so that she will be able to manage her own business matters.

A proud grandmother of six, Doris loves to keep active by dancing and taking long nature walks. An avid reader, she loves mysteries—and keeps sharp by trying to figure out the mystery herself. She'll put the book down and rerun the action in her mind until she has a solution to the situation.

"It helps," she says, "to think. I like to visualize into the distance what the place in the story looks like."

Doris prefers reading to watching stories on television, because she finds TV boring. "It's all mapped out for you. There's little to think about!"

need to exercise *all* areas of your brain. We will incorporate activities throughout the book to help you exercise all sections of your brain.

SEEK AND FIND PUZZLE

Here is a vocabulary activity that uses some of the words we define in this book. This puzzle is in the familiar Seek and Find format. Find the words in the array of letters inside the "brain." The words may appear spelled forward or backward, up or down, as well as diagonally. When you find them, circle them or use a highlighter to identify them.

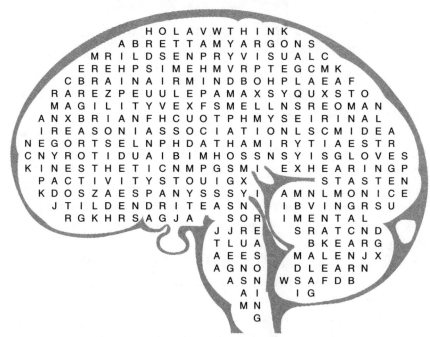

Seek and Find Word List

ACTIVITY	ESTROGEN	LEARN	SIGHT
AGELESS	EXERCISE	MEMORY	SMELL
AGILITY	GRAY	MENTAL	SPATIAL
ASSOCIATION	MATTER	MIND	SYNAPSE
AUDITORY	HEARING	MNEMONIC	TASTE
AXON	HEMISPERE	NEURON	TOUCH
BRAIN	HIPPOCAMPUS	PHYSICAL	VERBAL
CELLS	IDEA	REASONING	VISUAL
DENDRITE	KINESTHETIC	SENSORY	

The answer to this puzzle is on page 58.

SELF-QUIZ

In Chapters 1 and 2, you learned a great deal about how you learn and what your strengths are for acquiring new information. Let's take a moment to rehearse that knowledge. With this chapter, we introduce the self-quiz, a mechanism for organizing new knowledge and promoting long-term storage of it.

 # 1–2, Check the response most like you:

1. My preferred style for learning is
   _____ auditory _____ visual _____ kinesthetic.
2. A secondary style I can use is
   _____ auditory _____ visual _____ kinesthetic.

 # 3–5, Write in the blank.

3. An activity to increase proficiency in the third learning style might be _____
   _____
4. The nerve cells in my brain are called _____.
   (Hint: see page 21)
5. The message pathways that are created in my brain as I learn are called _____. (Hint: see page 21)

 # 6, Check the responses most like you:

6. Of the seven multiple intelligences, my expertise lies in all of the following:
   _____Linguistic
   _____Musical
   _____Logical-Mathematical
   _____Spatial
   _____Bodily-Kinesthetic
   _____Personal
   _____Naturalist

 # 7, Write in the blank:

7. An activity I might choose to increase my ability in one of the areas of multiple intelligences that at this time I do not possess would be _____
_____.

Answer to the Seek and Find puzzle:

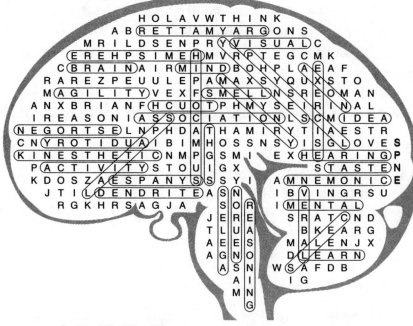

Seek and Find Word List

ACTIVITY	ESTROGEN	LEARN	SIGHT
AGELESS	EXERCISE	MEMORY	SMELL
AGILITY	GRAY	MENTAL	SPATIAL
ASSOCIATION	MATTER	MIND	SYNAPSE
AUDITORY	HEARING	MNEMONIC	TASTE
AXON	HEMISPERE	NEURON	TOUCH
BRAIN	HIPPOCAMPUS	PHYSICAL	VERBAL
CELLS	IDEA	REASONING	VISUAL
DENDRITE	KINESTHETIC	SENSORY	

REFERENCES:

1. Peter S. Eriksson et al. "Neurogenesis in the Adult Human Hippocampus," *Nature Medicine* (November 1998, 4 Number 11): 1313–1317.
2. J. Madeline Nash, "Special Report: Fertile Minds From Birth, A Baby's Cells Proliferate Wildly, Making Connections That May Shape a Lifetime of Experience," *Time*, 3 (February 1997): 48.
3. Robert Kunzig, "Climbing Through the Brain," *Discover Magazine*, 1 (August 1998): 60.
4. "Neuron Migration and Brain Disorders," *Brain Briefings* (January 1995); Marcia Barinaga, "Neurobiology: Researchers Find Signals that Guide Young Brain Neurons," *Science*, 17 (October 1997); Sharon Begley, "Your Child's Brain," *Newsweek*, 19 (February 1996): 55.
5. Kunzig, "Climbing Through the Brain."
6. Carla Shatz, "The Developing Brain," *Scientific American* (September 1992): 61.
7. "Neuron Migration and Brain Disorders," *Brain Briefings* (January 1995).
8. J. Madeline Nash, "Special Report: Fertile Minds From Birth, A Baby's Cells Proliferate Wildly, Making Connections That May Shape a Lifetime of Experience," *Time*, 3 (February 1997): 48.
9. Joel Davis, *Mapping the Mind. The Secrets of the Human Brain and How it Works* (Secaucus: Birch Lane Press, 1997); Carla Shatz, "The Developing Brain," *Scientific American* (September 1992): 61.
10. Sandra Ackerman, *Discovering the Brain* (Washington: National Academy Press, 1992).
11. Silvia Cardoso, "Neurons: Our Internal Galaxy," *Brain and Mind* (November 1998).
12. Sally P. Springer and Georg Deutsch, *Left Brain. Right Brain. Perspectives from Cognitive Neuroscience* (New York: W.H. Freeman and Company, 1998).

13. Doreen Kimura, "Sex, sexual orientation and sex hormones influence human cognitive function," in *Findings and Current Opinions in Cognitive Neuroscience*, ed. Larry Squire and Stephen Kosslyn (London: MIT Press, 1998); Anne Moir and David Jessel, *Brain Sex* (New York: Carol Publishing Group, 1991).
14. Silvia Cardoso, "The External Architecture of the Brain," *Brain and Mind* (March–May 1997).
15. Press release, University of Toronto, April 1, 1999.
16. Howard Gardner, *Frames of Mind. The Theory of Multiple Intelligences* (New York: Basic Books, 1993).
17. Oliver Koenig and Stephen Kosslyn, *Wet Mind: The New Cognitive Neuroscience* (New York: Free Press, 1995).
18. Michael D. Lemonick, "Glimpses of the Mind," *Time*, 17 (July 1995): 44.
19. Joel Davis, *Mapping the Mind. The Secrets of the Human Brain and How it Works* (Secaucus: Birch Lane Press, 1997).
20. Carla Shatz, "The Developing Brain," *Scientific American* (September 1992): 61.
21. Howard Gardner, *Frames of Mind. The Theory of Multiple Intelligences* (New York: Basic Books, 1993).
22. Carla Shatz, "The Developing Brain," *Scientific American* (September 1992): 61.
23. Gardner, *Frames of Mind*.
24. Doreen Kimura, "Sex, sexual orientation and sex hormones influence human cognitive function," in *Findings and Current Opinions in Cognitive Neuroscience*, ed. Larry Squire and Stephen Kosslyn (London: MIT Press, 1998).
25. Gardner, *Frames of Mind*.
26. Oliver Koenig and Stephen Kosslyn, *Wet Mind: The New Cognitive Neuroscience* (New York: Free Press, 1995).

27. Oliver Koenig and Stephen Kosslyn, *Wet Mind: The New Cognitive Neuroscience* (New York: Free Press, 1995).
28. "Memory Building," *The Economist*, 29 (August 1998).

Chapter

3

Teach Your Brain Agility

Engineer Your Own Learning

KEY CONCEPTS

Environmental Effects on Learning
Emotional Effects on Learning
Social Effects on Learning
Gender Differences and Learning

INTRODUCTION

In Chapter 1, you determined your preferences for acquiring information: visually, auditorially, or kinesthetically. In Chapter 2, you learned more than you probably ever wanted to know about how your brain processes the information you obtain. Now one more aspect of the learning process, and you will be fully prepared to tackle the techniques and strategies we present in the following chapters. A complete understanding allows you to control your own learning processes in day-to-day living and the learning you will be experiencing as you read this book.

Not only do you have information-delivery sensory preferences, you have environmental, emotional, and sociological preferences.[1] These characteristics are controlled by the *reticular system* (physical needs and immediate environment), the

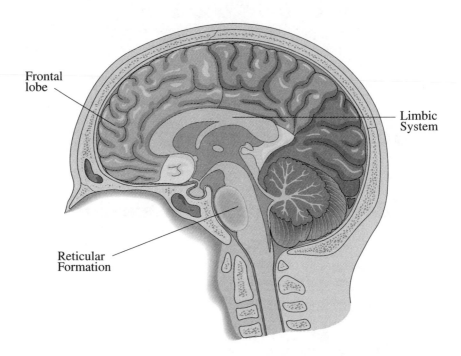

Frontal lobe

Limbic System

Reticular Formation

Figure 3-1 Control areas for environmental, emotional and sociological preferences

limbic system (emotionality), and the *frontal lobe* (sociological needs) of the brain (see Figure 3-1). For example, the reticular system functions to allow us to ignore distractions and concentrate on the task at hand. It is the subsystem used to ignore surrounding noises. It then causes us to pay attention to the noise when it changes. The limbic system is considered the source of emotional responses, and the frontal lobe has already been discussed in Chapter 2 as the seat of our knowledge of self.[2]

ENVIRONMENTAL EFFECTS

Your physical preferences include presentation styles, such as the size and legibility of the printed material, pitch or loudness of voices, and comfortable clothes in which to practice. Sometimes we can't remember things, or we remember them incorrectly, because of the quality of the presentation. For example, if the person's voice who is giving you an address to remember is pitched too low or they mumble, you may not hear the address or you may interpret it incorrectly. Likewise, struggling to read small print may reduce your efficiency when storing material.

Whatever you need to do to reduce the drain on your energies and allow yourself to be more efficient in a learning situation, do it. Here are some strategies others have found successful:

- Try large-print books. If the book is not available in large print, some folks have purchased a handheld magnifying glass or bought reading glasses.

- Try books on tape. You can adjust the volume, and professional speakers have very clear, precise speech.

- If the problem is an auditory one, ask people to speak more clearly or to talk louder.

- Some people need to practice something by writing it down. You might try this technique. To help, you might begin to carry a small notebook in your pocket or purse.

We all feel that time is too precious to waste! We can be efficient with our learning strategies. If we absorb the information accurately the first time, we can save ourselves stress and worry. Let's find the fastest, most effective learning methods for you. After all, if we don't remember something important, we will be the one who suffers.

Don't spend time being frustrated by something that can be corrected.

Circadian Rhythms

The time of day affects your ability to function. This is a result of your personal biological rhythms. *Circadian rhythms* are cycles with a period of about one day.[3] Biological rhythms, especially the Circadian rhythm, are discussed in more detail in Chapter 6, "Regain an Agile Brain." You may describe yourself as a morning person, or you may recognize that you are most energetic in the afternoon. Circadian rhythms are becoming increasingly important in the medical field as studies indicate that matching medicinal administration, surgery, and cancer treatments to your circadian rhythm increases the success and survival rate.[4] One example of the circadian rhythm is that many individuals find their energy level to be at its lowest after lunch. In fact, in traditional Mexican cultures, a siesta is a normal part of their routine. We often assume this is a result of eating. But our energy level does not drop after eating breakfast or supper, so this may be a result of your particular circadian rhythm. Because of circadian rhythms, there are variations in learning readiness as well. Some studies indicate that as we grow older, we begin to prefer the morning hours when energy is at a peak. But this is not true for everyone; others' energies may peak in the evening.[5]

Try to identify your time periods of peak performance. Schedule doctor visits or other important meetings when you are at your energy peak. Luncheons with business associates, relatives, or friends may be better rescheduled to breakfasts or dinners. You want to be at your best when interacting with others—not only because you want to leave a good impression, but also because it will help you to interact mentally at a higher performance level.

A note about circadian rhythms: It is difficult to be sympathetic with someone who is two or three rhythms different from you. It takes patience and understanding to realize that this is a natural pattern, not an indication of another person's lethargy or excitability!

Circadian Rhythms Quiz

This assessment instrument can help you identify your circadian rhythms. Place a check next to the items in each category that are most like you.

Sleep Habits

1. _____ I like to go to bed early, right after supper.
2. _____ I like to go to sleep in the early evening.
3. _____ I like to go to bed in mid-evening.
4. _____ I like to go to bed after the late news.
5. _____ I like to stay up late most of the time.
6. _____ I am a night owl. I catch up on my sleep in the daytime.

Waking Habits

1. _____ If I set the alarm clock for 7 A.M. or earlier, I often wake up before it goes off.
2. _____ I like to get up about 9 A.M. or 10 A.M.
3. _____ If I can sleep in, I usually wake up about 11 A.M.
4. _____ I could sleep all morning.
5. _____ I feel groggy if I have to get up before noon.
6. _____ Wake me about 2 P.M.

Mental Peaks

1. _____ I think best when I first get up in the morning.
2. _____ I tend to do my best thinking in the midmorning.
3. _____ Luncheon meetings are my best time to get things done.
4. _____ I am at my best in the afternoon.
5. _____ I put off weighty decisions to the evening hours.
6. _____ Late-night hours are my most creative and productive.

Energy Rhythms

1. _____ I wake up early and whistle or sing while getting dressed.

2. _____ I start to get going about 10 A.M.

3. _____ If I'm up in the morning, not much gets done. But at lunchtime, I come alive.

4. _____ I get a surge of energy in the afternoons.

5. _____ I tend to make appointments for evenings, because I have the most energy then.

6. _____ I would really like to work at night and be home during the day.

You may have noticed a pattern to the answer options. All responses to number 1 indicate that you function best in the early morning, 2 in the late morning, 3 midday, 4 midafternoon, 5 early evening, and 6 late at night.

In learning situations, many people want silence in order to concentrate, while others prefer background noise such as music. With the passing of years, a natural preference for background noise may interfere with our ability to learn as our hearing becomes less acute. If you are trying to concentrate and someone is making too much noise, ask that person to be a little quieter. Try earplugs if you need quiet.

Other Environmental Effects

Other environmental factors that affect our ability to process and retain information are temperature and light. If the surrounding temperature is too high or too low, we are uncomfortable, irritable, easily distracted, and our ability to concentrate lessens. As we age, we require better lighting in order to see more clearly. Proper illumination allows us to see a speaker's lips to assist our hearing, to read more easily and more quickly, and to perform tasks more accurately.

When you are experiencing difficulty concentrating, whether to memorize something or to recall something, check out your environment. Is the temperature comfortable or the light bright enough? Are there too many distractions? Are you struggling to hear or read? Do you need to move around or find a pencil and paper to doodle? You need to accommodate your natural preferences and requirements in order to operate more efficiently. Even if something you want to do seems silly to others, do it. Wouldn't you rather learn what you need to know?

EMOTIONAL EFFECTS

Mental abilities decrease more in people who experience negative emotions, such as depression, anxiety, bitterness, and anger, than in those who are happy or content with their lives. Robert Sapolsky, author of *Stress, the Aging Brain and the Mechanisms of Neuron Death*, theorizes that stress-related release of adrenal hormone bathes the neurons and eventually can damage the brain.[6]

Some of emotion's effects on the brain are merely distracting. Here are a few examples of those effects:

- Depression affects your motivation to remember, your ability to concentrate, and your perception of circumstances. It also can cause overreaction to slight lapses in memory.

- Moving to a new home can cause feelings of loneliness, grief, and an inability to concentrate.

- Retirement sometimes creates feelings of a lack of purpose, sadness, and a sense of loss.

- Often as we age, anxiety, loneliness, depression, and feelings of a lack of purpose increase.

These negative emotions cause us to disengage from life. Older adults should indeed become more concerned with the quality of life in their golden years. But they should not remove themselves from activities. Better that they recenter on what is important. Once we begin to withdraw from contact with others (perhaps because of ill health, a change in finances, moving to another location, or loss of a spouse), it is difficult to force ourselves to resume social interactions. People who regularly and actively engage in social interactions have better overall health and well-being than those who do not. And inactivity combined with little or no social contact diminishes or eliminates the need to exercise those brain cells and to practice remembering.

First, get a checkup to eliminate any physical reason for negative emotions. Then try to get busy. Here are some suggestions:

- Join a support group.
- Enroll in interesting classes.
- Make a new friend and learn something new together.
- Interact!

Work to improve your outlook on life. It will improve your mental capabilities as well!

SOCIAL EFFECTS

Your personality and sense of responsibility affect not only your relationships with others, your job, and your hobbies, but also your learning abilities and style. Some people are very self-driven. They are more likely to be lifelong learners. Many tend to be independent learners and do not require structured classes with instructors to guide them. Other individuals are peer-oriented and often follow the lead of another in unfamiliar situations. They are more likely to benefit from the assistance of a formal teaching environment. They may be less likely to pursue learning throughout life without direct access to formal learning scenarios or the influence of a friend or spouse.

It is vital to your health and longevity to remain a lifelong learner. Research studies indicate that lifelong learners tend to take better care of themselves, to be more aware of current health issues and breakthroughs, and to show an increase in IQ.[7] The increased IQ is extremely pertinent to you. In fact, a study of identical twins demonstrated that when one twin had a noticeably higher IQ score, that twin *always* lived longer.[8]

People who are more intelligent tend to live longer than people who are less intelligent.

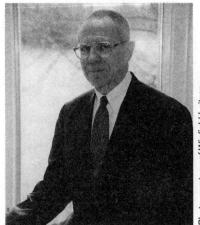

Photo courtesy of Winfield Leitzer

Older and Wiser

Bob Gifford, D.Ed., 79, was recruited into a volunteer program after retiring from 27 years with the county school system. He joined a group of enterprising people who helped other seniors prepare their income-tax returns in a program jointly sponsored by the American Association of Retired Persons (AARP) *and the local Department of Aging. Eventually, Bob became the countywide coordinator of the program. He was busy recruiting volunteers, training them, managing paperwork, and reporting to the sponsoring organizations. Bob says that he found the work as challenging as his assignments in the workforce. The frequent changes in tax laws and the unique tax-related situations of many of the seniors kept him learning new things.*

Bob spends the rest of the year working on other community projects. So much so that the local elementary school created a fitness trail and dedicated it in the names of Bob and his wife Rita. Now to keep up with two active grandchildren who live several states away, Bob is learning to use a computer. He quips, "Surely e-mail is only the tip of our learning curve as we get acquainted with the full potential of cyberspace."

Because most IQ tests measure your linguistic, mathematical, spatial, and logical deduction capabilities, start exercising those areas of your brain. If you don't want to take a formal class, use some word puzzle books, increase your vocabulary, start writing your life story, do logic puzzles, draw, paint, brush up on your math skills. Increase your intelligence. Increase the quality of your life.

GENDER DIFFERENCES

Our culture acknowledges equal opportunity for both sexes. However, the sexes are not equal. Some physical differences show up even before we are born. Gender differences are caused by the effects of both genes and hormones on the developing fetus. (See Chapter 2 for more details regarding the development of the prenatal child.) Genes alone do not determine the sex of a child. Appropriate hormonal levels must be present to ensure the proper growth of the fetus. These levels affect the internal wiring of the brain. For example, research indicates that individuals may have the chromosomes of a male, but without the necessary bathing of the fetus with male hormones at each of three critical periods during gestation, the child may appear physically female or may not be as traditionally masculine as expected.[9]

From the time of birth, males and females exhibit different preferences and abilities. In general, men see better in bright light, and women see better in the dark. Women are more sensitive to changes in pitch. As an example, when a woman begins to be annoyed, most of the other women in the room will know this immediately by the tone of her voice. However, the majority of men will not be aware of her annoyance until the change in pitch is much more pronounced. It is not that they are not paying attention or ignoring the annoyed woman's signals; they just do not detect the slight variations as well as women do. The following table lists a few of the other common differences.[10]

Men	Women
See in a narrow field	Greater peripheral vision
Greater depth perception	Less depth perception
More sensitive to saltiness	More sensitive to sweets Greater preference for sweets
Better hand-eye coordination Better at spatial abilities, such as constructing 3D objects from a flat design	Better at reading facial features Prefer to turn a map so that it is oriented in the same direction as they are traveling
Give directions using north, south, etc.	Give directions using visual cues, such as "turn right, there'll be a white house on the corner"
Better at abstract mathematical theories and relationships (better at story problems)	Better at algebraic processes such as adding, dividing, etc.
More prone to verbal difficulties; almost all people who stutter are male	Better verbal abilities
4 out of 5 dyslexics are male	Learn to read and write faster Find it easier to master foreign languages

These differences in preferential skills and abilities begin to be noticeable soon after birth and continue into adulthood. These preferences affect our abilities to notice details and to communicate in our personal and professional lives; they even affect the strategies we use to achieve success in our choice of goals. These differences between the sexes do not make one sex better than the other. We are different and complement each other. As the French say, "Viva la difference!"

SELF-QUIZ

Were you aware of the many factors affecting your mental abilities? Let's take a few moments to review your lifestyle and preferences.

Circadian Rhythms

What time of day do you feel your energy. level is highest? Color in the times of day and night that you are most energized. Use the clocks shown.

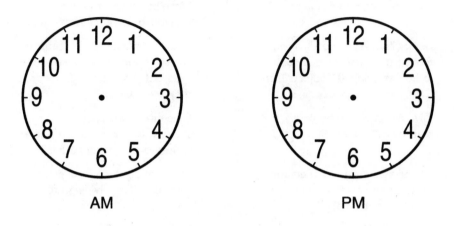

Color in the times of day and night that you have the least energy. Use the following clocks.

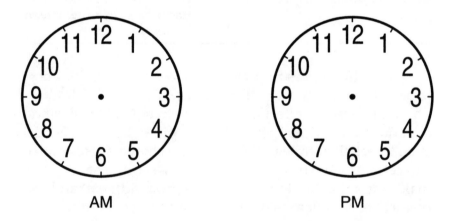

Note these times. Perhaps you can reschedule activities that require high levels of mental capability to those times.

Distractions

Choose from the following list those items that are most like you.

1. _____ I am not distracted very easily. When I concentrate, it's hard to interrupt me.

2. _____ Some noises interrupt my train of thought, such as these: _____

   _____.

3. _____ I am easily distracted. I can do the following to minimize distractions while I'm trying to think:

   _____

   _____.

When attempting to perform a task or remember a piece of information, distractions or background noise may make you forget where you were or what you were trying to remember. Start at the beginning and try again. Try to notice whether you forget what you're doing with or without distractions present. Be confident. It may not be memory lapses. Perhaps you simply got distracted from the task at hand.

Remembering

Notice what type of information you are concerned about forgetting. Be specific about what's bothering you. For example, "Have I always been forgetful about meeting times or places? Names? Messages?"

List a few problem areas

1. _____

2. _____

3. _____

After you identify a problem area, try to decide why you've changed (unless you determine that you have always been forgetful!).

List some reasons why these areas you wrote about have become a problem:

1. _____
2. _____
3. _____

If you're worrying about becoming senile, ask others. Ask your friends. Ask them whether you seem to be forgetting more often than before.

Here are some questions you can ask about remembering:

1. _____ Is the importance of remembering less acute?
2. _____ Has job pressure been reduced?
3. _____ Have I retired and am now "relaxing" too much?
4. _____ Did I pay enough attention to the information when I encountered it?
5. _____ Am I grieving over the loss of a loved one?
6. _____ Do I miss lost friends due to a recent move?

Here are some explanations that might help you understand some of the reasons you were forgetting things. Perhaps you lost a spouse to death or divorce, and you were in the habit of depending on that spouse to remember things for you. Grief may cause you to become more easily distracted. Often, when you think you forgot something, or you're accused of forgetting something, you simply did not pay enough attention to pass the information successfully to long-term memory and then create an association to retrieve it. Most information never makes it to long-term memory. Not paying adequate attention accounts for approximately 50 percent of reported memory problems. However, not only do you need to get the information successfully transferred to long-term memory, but you must be able to retrieve it. Thus, you need an incentive to make it worthwhile to concentrate, store the information, and create an association to retrieve it. The incentive may be job security, pride, or health, for example.

Chapter 4, "Develop a Brawny Brain," discusses various strategies you can use to reinforce your current learning techniques. Applications and games using various strategies are provided so that you can practice new techniques and refine old ones to improve and maintain your mental agility.

REFERENCES:

1. Rita Dunn and Kenneth Dunn. *Teaching Secondary Students Through Their Individual Learning Styles* (Boston: Allyn and Bacon, 1992).
2. Howard Gardner, *Frames of Mind. The Theory of Multiple Intelligences* (New York: Basic Books, 1993).
3. Lynne Lamberg, "A Matter of Time," *BrainWork* (March/
April 1998): 6.
4. Isadora Stehlin, "A Time to Heal: Chronotherapy Tunes in to Body's Rhythms," *FDA Consumer*, 1 (April 1997, 31).
5. Roy Shephard. *Aging, Physical Activity, and Health* (Champaign, IL.: Human Kinetics, 1997).
6. Robert Sapolsky, *Stress, the Aging Brain, and the Mechanisms of Neuron Death* (MIT Press, 1992).
7. Daniel Golden, "Building a Better Brain," *Life* (July 1994): 63.
8. K. Warner Schaie, Ph.D., *Adult Development and Aging* (Harper Collins, 1991), 415.
9. Doreen Kimura, "Sex Differences in the Brain," *Scientific American* (September 1992).
10. Anne Moir and David Jessel, *Brain Sex* (New York: Carol Publishing Group, 1991).

C h a p t e r

4

Develop a Brawny Brain

Build a Mental Agility
Exercise Program

KEY CONCEPTS

Distractions and Attention
Information-Storing Preferences
Information-Retrieval Strategies
Information-Processing Activities

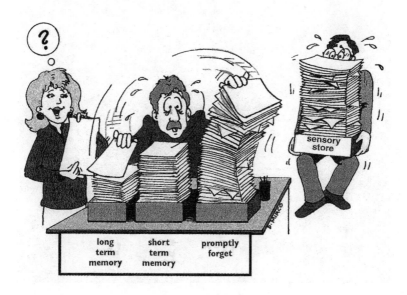

INTRODUCTION

You learned in earlier chapters how exercising your brain can improve your intellectual ability. In this chapter, we'll introduce you to basic storage and retrieval techniques that you can use as part of your mental-agility exercise program. More advanced variations of these techniques and exercises are presented in greater detail in Chapters 6, "Regain an Agile Brain," and 7, "Enjoy Your Ageless Mental Agility."

Mental exercises can take many forms: brain teasers, games, puzzles, bridge, going back to school, and more. Learning something new, whether in a formal school setting or independently, is an excellent exercise. Distinct areas of the brain are activated as you graduate from a novice to a more experienced level in mastery of a technique or subject. Figure 4-1 is a PET scan that demonstrates the various areas of the brain that are energized and exercised when a linguistic technique is introduced. The subject is observed while still a novice and unpracticed, versus when he or she is experi-

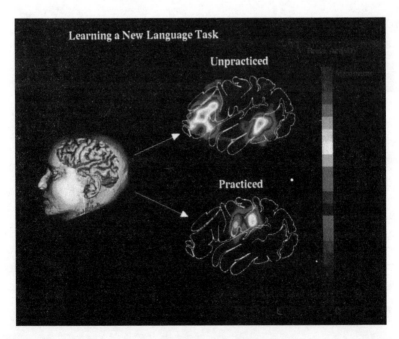

Figure 4-1 PET scan of brain activity of novice compared to expert

enced and practiced. Notice that as you become familiar with a topic, the area of the brain being used will change. Remember from the first two chapters, though, that the areas of the brain that are activated depend on what you are learning and how you are going about learning it.

Remember when you last learned something new? Perhaps it was learning a new dance step, making a new recipe, or trying to use a new piece of equipment. Try to think of that last thing you learned. Check as many as apply to you.

Did you have to:

_____ Learn new words?

_____ Memorize anything?

_____ Look up information?

_____ Ask someone for information?

_____ Practice anything?

_____ Explain what you learned to someone else?

Was it:

_____ Hard to learn?

_____ Not so hard to learn?

_____ Easy to learn?

Were you:

_____ Fascinated?

_____ Fearful?

_____ Fine?

Initially, you probably had to exert a lot of effort and concentration. People who are learning a new dance step, for example, find that it takes a great deal of concentration at the beginning. As you mastered the topic of interest, you likely required less conscious effort. Notice in Figure 4-1 how the PET scan demonstrates a decrease in the energy required to perform the task as the subject became more expert and comfortable with the technique. The subject's brain became more efficient—the same as your brain becomes more efficient as you become more expert.

As you became more interested in the subject, did you talk to other people about your newest interest and get their input? Perhaps you searched out information to make you more knowledgeable in the same topic or a related one. The benefits are quite broad. By talking to others, you exercise other areas of your brain, such as the intrapersonal or linguistic area. You also might have branched into other areas, such as the right hemisphere for a touch of imagination to become more innovative, or perhaps tapped into your spatial abilities.

In this section of the book, we are going to present various strategies to process information and learn something new. Be aware that by practicing these techniques in a learning situation, you are exercising many regions of the brain. You might feel rusty in the beginning, but remember that as you practice, the activity shifts into other areas of the brain, and you become more efficient as you become more practiced and relaxed. You wouldn't want to exercise only one area of your body, so be sure that you practice all the following techniques in various types of learning situations and exercise all of your brain. Also be sure to discuss and practice these techniques with your friends and family and exercise those linguistic, intrapersonal, and interpersonal skills.

INFORMATION PROCESSING

Information processing describes an active method for learning something new. It is very easy to allow new information to pass us by. It takes a dynamic analysis of the information to make sense of it—to move it from short-term to long-term memory. You must make the new information meaningful for your brain so that the ideas will become important enough to make their way to long-term memory. In this chapter, you will learn how to work with information so that you can better remember it.

When we were young, we preferred to use one hand more often than the other. Over time, we became skilled with that hand and rarely used the other hand except for balance or coordination with our dominant hand. We can perform gross motor skills with the other hand, such as opening a door or petting an animal. Without thinking about it, we simply use our dominant hand. Some people who have lost function in their dominant hand find that, with practice, they can become facile with their less-dominant hand. Their handwriting may never be as clear with the new hand, but it can be understood.

So it is with our preferred learning styles. Early on, we all found the best way for us to learn and, without thinking about it, applied that style to every situation. In Chapter 1, you learned what your dominant learning preference is, while in Chapter 2, you evaluated your natural intelligences. In this chapter you will explore supplementary ways to learn and how to develop your less-dominant learning styles and increase your use of the other intelligences. This information will provide you with a wide spectrum of fresh tricks to use when trying to learn something new!

You can assess your current information-processing skills before reading this chapter by taking the preassessment that follows. Then, after reading about how to learn more efficiently and practicing your new skills, you may reassess your processing ability with the postassessment at the end of this chapter.

INFORMATION-PROCESSING PREASSESSMENT

Directions: Read the following paragraphs. Then answer 10 questions about the information regarding Figure 4-2.

Suppose you are going to run some errands. You should drive to these places, because some have drive-in windows and you will have much to carry. You need to take six shirts and a suit to the cleaners, pick up shoes at the shoe repair, and get two birthday cards at the drugstore where you have to pick up a prescription.

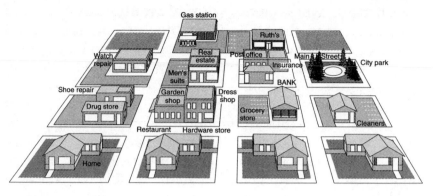

Figure 4-2

Your wristwatch is repaired and ready for pickup. You also need to get bread, ice cream, bananas, rice, and soup at the grocery store. You made a list, but somehow it got lost along the way. Your sister is waiting for you to pick her up at Ruth's beauty shop. You'd better get going. The bank closes at 2:30 today, and you have to deposit your check.

Now answer the following questions, being sure not to look back at the information just reviewed.

Questions

1. What do you need at the grocery store?_____
   _____

2. Who is waiting at the beauty shop? _____

3. Did you need to go to the post office? _____

4. What is the name of the beauty shop owner? _____
   _____

5. What do you need to drop off at the cleaners? _____
   _____

6. What other places do you need to visit?_____
   _____

7. Which is closer to the post office, the bank or the drug-store? _____

8. What do you need from the hardware store? _____
_____

9. Do you need to drop off the shoes at the shoe repair?
_____

10. What do you need at the drugstore?_____
_____

After you complete the questionnaire, check your answers at the end of this chapter in "Solutions to Exercises and Games."

This is a very difficult exercise. Don't be discouraged if you couldn't answer every question. In the following sections, you will learn techniques for improving your ability to work with exercises similar to these. Move ahead with the notion that you are collecting new tools, looking for new ways to a solution, and listening for new tips.

DISTRACTIONS AND ATTENTION

It is vitally important to the learning process that we pay attention and do not allow ourselves to be distracted from the information we are trying to process. We are trying to get this information from *short-term memory* (STM) to *long-term memory* (LTM), and this requires the brain to restructure. (See Chapter 2 for details.)

Let's take, for example, the seemingly simple but amazingly complex task of learning another person's name as we are introduced. Many people are quite eager (and seemingly proud) to announce that they cannot remember people's names even if they have just been introduced. They can acknowledge that an introduction has taken place, but they have no recollection of the name of the person. Often, the problem is easy to diagnose. At the instant of an introduction, the person's name is in the sensory store. We should be making efforts to pass the person's name to STM and on to LTM. And indeed we are concentrating, but not necessarily on the name. Pressures in our culture divert our attention from the person we are meeting. This distraction may arise from our need to present ourselves well and make a good impression during the introduction. We also may be trying to be polite and pay attention to what the other person is saying. The little niceties and good manners are taking our attention away from the information we want to save. Whatever the reason, many people do not move the new person's name from the sensory store to LTM simply because they have not paid enough attention to exactly what they want to transfer. This is one example of intense concentration used incorrectly.

There are strategies to help you pay more attention at the moment of the introduction. You might use your preferred learning style to help learn the name. If you are a visual learner, you might want to visualize the name on a theater marquee. Asking a woman about the spelling of her name gives more attention to the name. For example, there are a va-

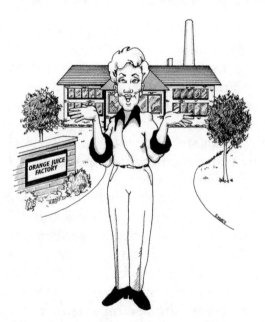

Tillie finally retired from the orange juice factory. She just couldn't concentrate.

riety of ways to spell Kathy: Cathy, Kathi, Cathie, and others. An auditory learner might want to repeat the person's name aloud or find a rhyme to the name. One of our friends uses *pretzel* to remind him of *Wetzel*. Linking the name to a physical object helps kinesthetic learners. A name such as *Harmeyer* contains an *arm* and an *eye*. Looking for these 3D representations of a name helps a kinesthetic learner pay attention.

Once you have your attention focused on a person, it may help to create a mental picture of the person. Associating her name with another person or group will help. For example, if her name is common, link it to people with the same or similar names whom you already know. Using the person's name as soon as possible and often during the first conversation will help you store the name. However, too much of a good thing might annoy your new acquaintance. So go easy!

If you realize that you are easily distracted, and you know the introduction is coming, you can start noticing characteristics of the person as you walk over. Practice the name and the mechanisms you are going to use to remember the name after the conversation is over and you are moving away from each other. In other words, *you* select as much as possible the time you are concentrating in order to avoid as many distractions as possible. You also might tell people at the end of the conversation that you are learning to remember names and give your own name again. People usually are relieved and repeat their own name as you say your good-byes. You can practice as you leave and are less distracted by the conversation.

You may not feel that introductions are the most important concern in your life. And indeed, they may not be unless you are very active socially or introductions are a business concern. But regardless of the learning situation, you need to be in control as much as possible in order to limit the number of distractions as you try to process information. Remember the discussion in Chapter 3 regarding the environment and distractions? Be sure you are truly focusing on the material you want to transfer to LTM.

After the name gets into your brain, how can you be sure you can get it out when you need it at a later meeting? Reconstructing the scene where you learned her name may help jog your memory. Look carefully at her face in case you associated a feature with her name. Try not to get upset. Some enzymes block your synaptic activity under stress. Give yourself enough time to recall her name. Don't set the goal that you must say "Hello . . . " using her name. If you relax, the name may come to you during the conversation, and you can use it then.

You can use these techniques for introductions in many other situations. Try to implement a few of these recommendations to help you concentrate. In the meantime, we have a few exercises for you to try.

 ## Visual Concentration

To improve your visual concentration, look at a scene in a room, outside, or in a magazine. Look for about 30 seconds, concentrating on what you see. At the end of the 30 seconds, turn away or close your eyes and try to remember everything you saw in the scene. Repeat this exercise with another scene. Practice this often. It's a good game to play while waiting for someone. Notice how your ability to recall more items in the scene improves as you play more often.

 ## Auditory Concentration

This is a game two or more people can play to develop their auditory concentration skills. It's called "I'm shopping!" To play, choose someone to go first. The first person says "I'm shopping for . . . " and names an object. The next person repeats what the first person says and adds a product. Keep playing while people can keep up with the complete list, and restart the game when someone forgets a product. Remember to have fun with this game. If someone who is playing forgets often, let that person go second. That way, the player can build on success more easily.

Kinesthetic Concentration

This is a game that will help you improve your concentration skills and have fun at the same time. You will need a regular deck of cards. Start with two suits: one red suit and one black suit. Add the two jokers. You will have 28 cards, two of each number and face card. Shuffle the cards. Place them face down in four rows of seven cards, as shown in Figure 4-3.

Turn over two cards at a time. If they are the same numbers, remove them from the game. If they are not the same numbers, remember what the numbers are, and turn them face down again. Continue until you have removed all pairs from the game. This game also can be played by two or more players. When one player fails to produce a pair, the next player takes over. As your concentration improves, add the rest of the deck to the game and draw four cards at a time. Visit the Web site associated with this book, www.mentalagility.com, to play an interactive version of this game.

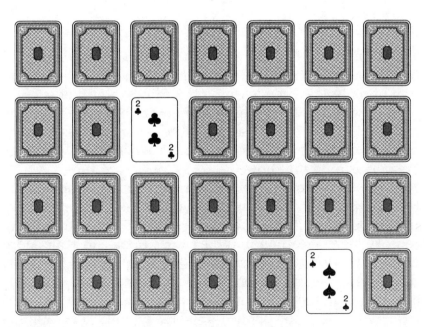

Figure 4-3 Kinesthetic Concentration Game

If you do not have a deck of cards, you might use dominos or 3-by–5–inch cards and write facts on them that you are trying to master.

INFORMATION-STORING PREFERENCES

Many people have developed clever strategies to help them learn new information. The following sections are structured so that you can discover new strategies. You may recognize some of them as ones you use already. In each of the sections, you will be told what skill you are exercising and how the activity will improve your ability to process information.

Researchers found that when the presentation of information and testing format match, performance increases. This means that if you are going to have to write something, practice writing; if you are going to have to say it, practice talking; if you are going to have to do something, practice doing it.

Rehearsal

The information-storing technique of *rehearsal* borrows its name from the theater. Actors and actresses use the repetition of material when learning their lines, aloud or silently, until they commit those lines to memory. Some people copy and then recopy the lines. The entire cast rehearses the play often so that everyone will remember what to do when they are performing the show.

You may have used rehearsal to remember a phone number by repeating it from the time you looked it up in the telephone book until you dialed it. This moved it from your sensory store—reading it in the phone book—to your short-term memory. The memory persisted long enough to let you dial the number. However, because it had no special meaning attached to it, the phone number didn't make it to *long-term memory (LTM)*. If the phone number is an important number (your mother's new telephone number, for example), you may want to take steps to promote its move to LTM. Re-

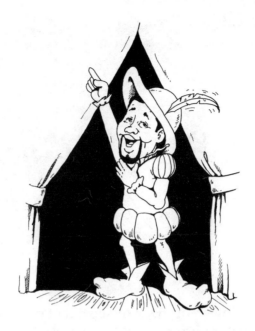

"To be at the doctor's appointment at 10:30 A.M. or not to be at the dinner party at 6:00 P.M."

hearsal can help. Reading the number over and over may help (visual learning style). Saying the number aloud repeatedly may help (auditory learning style). Writing the number repeatedly or dialing the number repeatedly also may help (kinesthetic learning style). You may discover that you use rehearsal techniques quite often. Some examples include directions to someone's home or business, items to purchase at the store, or errands to run.

Repetition Priming

Repetition priming is a technical phrase for what you have experienced if you can sing the jingle "See the USA in your Chevrolet!" or if you remember that Nancy Reagan wanted us to "Just Say No!" Repetition priming goes along with rehearsal because the repeated hearing or seeing of information increases your recall of that information. The repetition, however, may not be conscious. You may be unaware of the

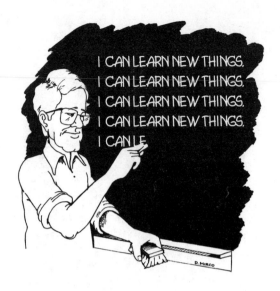

number of times you hear or see a fact or notion. This is the advantage of advertising. We remember what we hear and see over and over and over. You may need a map or a set of directions to visit a friend's home for the first time. After a few visits, however, you can find the way without the map or directions. You may not have made a conscious determination to learn the way to her home, but the repetition helped you learn the way.

A research study was performed in which tapes of word associations were played to patients who were anesthetized for surgery (with their prior consent). Testing later demonstrated that the patients had subliminally heard the tapes.[1] This test also demonstrates the importance of talking to patients who are unconscious, especially in an uplifting, encouraging manner. It also may explain why associating with someone who constantly belittles you can seep into your subconscious and then into your conscious mind, affecting your attitude toward yourself. If you are trying to learn a new language, it helps to play tapes of people speaking the language. You can turn this technique to your advantage.

Repetition Priming ADvantage

This game emphasizes the power of repetition priming. Write in the blank next to each slogan the name of the touted product. Check your answers at the end of this chapter in "Solutions to Exercises and Games."

1. It's 99 and $^{44}/_{100}$ percent pure _____

2. The foaming cleanser _____

3. Because I'm worth it _____

4. Just do it! _____

5. And away go troubles down the drain _____

6. Must-see TV _____

7. Mmm-mmm good! _____

8. The real mayonnaise _____

9. Fly the friendly skies. _____

10. When you care enough to send the very best _____

11. We do chicken right. _____

12. Put a tiger in your tank. _____

13. The breakfast of champions _____

14. Tony the tiger says it's GREAT! _____

15. 31 flavors _____

You may not have heard some of these slogans for many years; yet you recognize them and can match them with their products. The power of repetition priming is that your brain creates many connections to information from simply hearing it over and over and over.

To understand how powerful this repetition-priming mechanism is, repeat this exercise with the products you remembered and write down the *current* marketing slogans.

Did you notice that the older slogans are more easily recalled? That is the signature of repetition priming. Once you've "got it," the information, however valuable, is there for a very long time without a conscious effort at memorization on your part.

Imaging

If you are a visual learner, you probably create visual images automatically to help you remember information. The image may contain words or objects, but you can *see* the information in your mind. If your dominant learning style is not visual, you can learn to create these images. Practice on a grocery list. Try to learn the items on that list. Imagine yourself in the food store, walking down the aisles to locate the items. See yourself picking up an item and putting it into the grocery cart. Repeat this for each of the items.

When you get to the store, you may use visual images to "see" your kitchen and remember what you need to buy. Buying clothes for someone else, you use your visual/spatial abilities to imagine the person, his size, and how the shirt you are holding will fit and look on him. Looking at the plans for a new house or the pattern for a new dress also requires exercising your spatial capabilities.

For some people, distractions inhibit their ability to create images. Concentrate on the information so that it is in

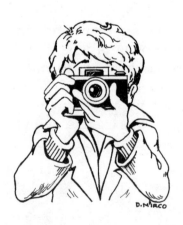

your sensory store. It helps to close your eyes and try to see the information in your mind. If a natural image does not present itself, create an image of your own. The more unusual the visual image, the more likely you will be able to recall it. Suppose that you are looking for a new car. You are trying to remember the features of one automobile over another. See each car in your mind with the features dancing in and out of the car.

If you are not accustomed to making a mental image whenever new information presents itself, this exercise will help you learn how to do that. For each of the following questions, try to imagine what the referenced object looks like. To increase your kinesthetic skill, move your body to respond to these questions. For example, if you are asked to identify the direction in which you turn a doorknob, use your hands to help create a mental image of yourself actually turning the knob. In each case, your creation of the mental image is far more important than the correct answer. However, for those of us who just need to know whether we are right, the answers are listed at the end of this chapter in "Solutions to Exercises and Games."

Imagine That

Create a mental picture to answer the following questions.

Imaging Questions

1. On the touch-tone telephone keypad, where is the # key?_____

2. On the head of a tiger, are the ears above, even with, or below the nose? _____

3. How many tines does a dinner fork have? _____
   _____

4. On each M&M's candy piece, there is a stamped letter. Is it a lowercase letter or an uppercase letter? _____
   _____

5. To turn on a lamp, do you turn the knob clockwise or counterclockwise? _____

6. To unlock a door, do you turn the key clockwise or counterclockwise? _____

7. To open a jar, do you twist the lid clockwise or counterclockwise? _____

8. Speaking of clocks, where is the hour hand at 7:30?
   _____

9. In what direction do you turn a light bulb to remove it?
   _____

10. On the waning moon, from the full moon to the new moon, which side of the moon is bright, the left or the right? _____

11. To open a door, in which direction do you turn the knob—toward the doorjamb or away from the doorjamb? _____

12. When you open a peanut shell, how many peanuts do you usually find? _____

13. At the dinner table, on what side of the plate is the knife? _____

14. Draw the symbol for a pharmacy. _____

15. On a computer keyboard or on a standard typewriter, where are the number keys? _____

16. On a hand calculator, is the 1 key on the top row of number keys or on the bottom? _____

17. On the telephone touch pad, is the 1 key on the top row of number keys or on the bottom? _____

18. On the ATM touch pad, is the 1 key on the top row of number keys or on the bottom? _____

19. In the alphabet, what is the first uppercase letter printed without a straight line? _____

20. In the alphabet, what is the last uppercase letter printed without a straight line? _____

If you have strong kinesthetic tendencies, you might have used your hands to help you visualize these situations.

If you have strong auditory tendencies, you might have read these sentences aloud to help you form visual images.

Coding

Coding is the creation of a mnemonic or catch phrase that associates material with something that is already familiar. The more complex the material, the more likely coding or imagery should be used as a memory technique.

Some people find success associating a list of items with a mnemonic device. In grade school, for example, we learned that the first letters of the Great Lakes could be rearranged to spell the word HOMES (Huron, Ontario, Michigan, Erie, and Superior). To remember the names, we just needed to remember HOMES. When we need to remember the names of the lakes, we also remember the mnemonic. We then can use it to reconstruct the original list. A link to a song or poem also is helpful. You may have learned the alphabet to the strains of *Twinkle, Twinkle Little Star* and the number of days in each month with the poem *30 Days Hath September.* Rosemary Austin, an intellectually active senior, remembers her license plate, 642 BBW, with the device that the numbers are reverse counting by twos and the letters represent Better Be Wary.

Connections that you make will be stored in your memory along with the ideas you are trying to remember. The more connections we have to a fact, the easier it is to retrieve it later. The curious thing about making associations with mnemonics is that the time and mental energy we put into developing them generally is enough prestorage processing that we tend to remember the original ideas. This extra concentration alerts the brain that this information is important, and with that added meaning, the memory is more likely to be stored permanently.

Demonic Mnemonics

In this exercise, you will practice decoding mnemonics. This should give you some ideas of how to create mnemonics of your own. Check your answers at the end of this chapter in "Solutions to Exercises and Games."

Match each mnemonic in the left column to its description in the right column. (Place the letter from column 2 in the blank next to its mnemonic.)

Mnemonic

1. ___ A rat in the house might eat the ice cream.

2. ___ ROY G BIV

3. ___ Say, I like a cuppa aspartame in drinks.

4. ___ Please excuse my dearAunt Sally.

5. ___ GAG SALE

6. ___ All animals play instruments.

7. ___ Some chaps think Da Vinci painted portraits and angels.

8. ___ When a jury makes miscreants angry, justice very happily triumphs.

9. ___ AAA goes Anywhere and Everywhere, North and South.

10. ___ Divorced, beheaded, died. divorced, beheaded, survived.[2]

Represented by Mnemonic

a. Order of operations on a hand calculator: parentheses, exponents, multiply and divide, add and subtract.

b. The fate of Henry VIII's six wives.

c. The choirs of angels: Seraphim, Cherubim, Thrones, Dominations, Virtues, Powers, Principalities, Archangels, and Angels.

d. 3.1415926, first eight digits of π.

e. Oceans of the world: Atlantic, Arctic, Pacific, and Indian.

f. Spelling of arithmetic.

g. Washington, Adams, Jefferson, Madison, Monroe, Adams, Jackson, Van Buren, Harrison, Tyler.

h. Colors of the rainbow: red, orange, yellow, green, blue, indigo, and violet.

i. The seven deadly sins: greed, avarice, gluttony, sloth, anger, lust, and envy.

j. The continents: Asia, Africa, Australia, Antarctica, Europe, North America, and South America.

Hierarchies

Making connections between bits of information tends to help us retrieve that information faster and more completely with less effort than that expended trying to recall disassociated memories. Organizing the memories into groups of people or things, by class, type, or rank helps to make more

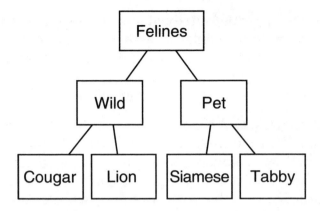

Figure 4-4 Animal hierarchy

connections. There is efficiency in hierarchies that help us make connections. Consider the feline family in Figure 4-4. There are similarities among the members of that group of animals. What we know about a lion, for example, tells us many things about a domestic pet: its coat is fur, its face has whiskers, its movement is sleek and silent, and more. By connecting a person or object with a group, we do not have to make a long list of details about the new object. We allow the object to inherit the qualities of the group, which we already have stored in our memories.

Many groups have an inherent ranking system. The Armed Forces, for example, are organized into a very structured ranking system where varying layers of officers take orders from and give orders to other soldiers in other strata in the ranks. In the Army, the generals are at the top. The succeeding ranks of commissioned officers include Colonel, Major, Captain, and Lieutenant. The higher the rank, the more privileges and the more responsibility the officer bears. There are common features to all of the ranks.

Rank Has Its Privilege

This exercise provides practice in your new skill of noting rank within a hierarchy.

Suppose that you are going to the grocery store and have to buy the following items: eggs, bread, lettuce, milk, broccoli, oranges, and sugar. Group the items in an upper level of a hierarchy. After you decide on a proper hierarchy for these foods, cover up this page and write the items in a list in the order you determined.

Solution: You could put them in a number of hierarchies.

1. You might use the groups formed by the Food Guide Pyramid in Figure 4-5. Sugar belongs at the top in the *use sparingly* category. Next, group the eggs and milk in the meat and dairy group. The third level is fruits and vegetables. Put broccoli, oranges, and lettuce in that group. The bottom of the pyramid is for breads. So, you need sugar, two meat and dairy, three fruit and vegetables, and one bread.

2. You might employ the hierarchy based on the layout of your grocery store. Group the items by the aisle in which they are stacked: milk and eggs at the dairy counter; lettuce, broccoli, and oranges in the produce aisle; bread in the bakery; and sugar in the seasoning aisle. So, you need two dairy, three produce, one bakery, and one seasoning.

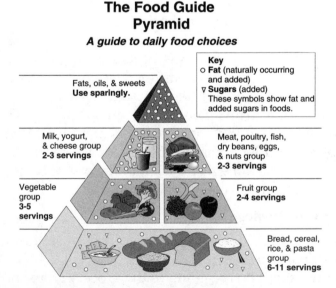

Figure 4-5 The Food Guide Pyramid

You may have decided on another appropriate hierarchy. The decision on a proper rank and then the arrangement of the items into that rank is the key to this new skill.

Determining the framework of the rank helps you concentrate more on the items in the list while you find an appropriate ranking scheme. That alone will aid you in trying to remember them.

Follow-up: Repeat this exercise with items you have on a shopping list in your home.

If It Looks Like a Duck and Walks Like a Duck . . .

This exercise provides practice in the notion that items in a hierarchy inherit properties from the higher-ranked objects. In the following game, you will practice identifying a common class to which a set of objects belong.

For each of the following collections, name a larger class to which all items belong:

1. _____ collies, schnauzers, scotties, retrievers

2. _____ cup, saucer, plate, bowl

3. _____ cat, dog, bird, hamster, guinea pig

4. _____ apple, aces, acre, ax, argyles

5. _____ bookkeeper, sleeper, Aaron, nook, muumuu, Hawaii

6. _____ Des Moines, Albany, Salem, Austin, Tallahassee

7. _____ turnip, carrot, beet, potato, rutabaga

8. _____ madam, radar, level, a Toyota, wow, Bob, noon

9. _____ knife, blade, scarf, purse, table

10. _____ birds, airplanes, angels, hospitals

11. _____ records, games, pianos, doctor, the stock market

12. _____ newspapers, tea leaves, palms, books, signs

13. _____ Humpty Dumpty, year, river, wig-maker

14. _____ refrigerator, nose, jogger, stockings

15. _____ envelopes, oceans, the president, *Good Housekeeping*™ magazine

Check your answers at the end of this chapter in "Solutions to Exercises and Games."

Follow-up: Now that you have the hang of it, make up collections of your own.

Follow-up: Play ANIMAL, a game of hierarchy. You can find this interactive game on the Ageless Mental Agility Web site at www.mentalagility.com. You can download the program to play with your family or play it online.

Chunking

Grouping items in a long list helps to reduce the number of items in the list. This technique is known as *chunking*. This helps to make a long list shorter, thereby reducing the number of items you need to remember. Chunking helps you remember telephone numbers. Each 10-digit telephone number is divided into three parts: the three-digit area code, the three-digit exchange office, and the four-digit line number. To remember a 10-digit telephone number, try chunking the area code and the exchange. Then you only have to remember the four-digit line number. For example, you can reduce the number 410–727–9416 to six items by remembering that 410 is a Maryland area code and 727 is a downtown Baltimore exchange. Recall only MD, Baltimore, 9416—six items! Now this won't help much in you live in an area other than Baltimore and don't know the area code and common exchanges to help you. You will have to personalize these examples in the book to match your situations.

Here is another example of chunking. For a Los Angeles phone number, you can chunk one of the area codes, 714, into Joe Friday's badge number from the detective show *Dragnet*. You also may chunk patterns in a telephone number. The number 202–555–1212 is directory assistance for Manhattan. Remember that 202 is a *palindrome* (the same number reading forward and backward), the exchange is all fives, and the line is two 12s. Remember that what we show are only examples. The brainwork necessary to adapt these exercises to your telephone area is good exercise!

INFORMATION-RETRIEVAL STRATEGIES

Information is power, but you must have the information when you need it. In fact, managing information systems is a major undertaking in any business. Keeping information

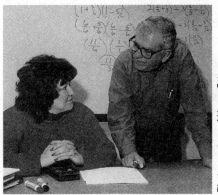

Photo courtesy of Henry Ortega

Older and Wiser

Mr. Salazar, age 73, had worked for 31 years as a petroleum engineer before retirement. He is widely known in Texas for his involvement in many diverse community development activities. Antonio is also extremely active in the Hispanic community and yet finds the time and energy to work part time teaching mathematics at a local community college. He takes great pride and pleasure in motivating his students, passing along to his students the techniques he used to learn, and keeping them advised of opportunities for advancement.

available for rapid retrieval is critical. Now that you have strategies to get the information into your brain, you need to develop a few strategies for getting the information back out in a timely manner.

At one time or another, you probably tried to reach a destination and encountered a roadblock. The availability of another route was critical to getting there. So it is with learning. Your brain stores information in distinct neural pathways. The more connections you make at the moments of learning, the more pathways are available to recover the fact when you need it. There are several techniques for doing so.

In geography class, you learned the names of the continents. You may have learned them in a pattern. You may have linked them by size. You may have linked them by hemispheres or by bodies of water. You may have memorized their positions on a globe. When asked to recite the list, you recalled them in the manner you stored them and listed their names.

Suppose that you are asked to list them in order of the number of letters in their names. Surely there is no connection in your brain for that order! You will need to use one of your other connections to recall all seven names and then process the list in a separate mental activity to arrive at the answer.

One of the best ways to create and fine-tune connections is to teach something to someone else. There is an old saying: *You never really understand something until you teach it.* You might want to consider using your skills and knowledge to help others learn. You get the benefits of reactivating the connections you made when you learned the material and the benefits of the new learner's view of the material. A prime example of passing along information strategies is Antonio Salazar.

Search Strategies

When a prompt for information and the connection to that information are present simultaneously, we call the phenomenon *instant recall.* The memory is triggered by the stimulation of the connection. Suppose that you need to recall

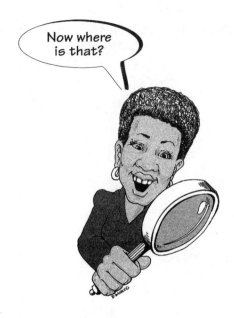

some information and it is not available instantly. Sometimes you try to remember something and can't. It's right on the tip of your tongue. You know you should be able to remember it, but you simply can't find the fact. You can use some retrieval strategies to locate a connection that does trigger the memory. Looking for the information you need is a skill you can master.

The following is a list of search strategies you can use to trigger that memory.

Alphabetic search	Recite the alphabet slowly. Perhaps the connection you are looking for is the first letter of the word.
Scenario search	Visualize the scene, the people, and the location where you learned the information.
Association search	Try to see, hear, or touch something that you originally associated with the fact.

Chronological search	Retrace your steps in time in order to locate the moment when you last used the fact.
Event search	What were you doing when you used the information?
Visual search	Try to see the paper on which the words were written.
People search	Recall the people with whom you used the information. What did they say or do or look like?
Increased stimulus search	Keep listening to the request or ask for more information. This one is hard to understand at first, but it is one of the most powerful.

Let's look at one example of how the increased stimulus search works. Consider this exchange:

Jane: You remember Janet, don't you?

Annette: No.

Jane: Sure you do. We met her while we were together.

Annette: No, but keep talking to see if you can jog my memory.

Jane: OK, we were at the Red Cross luncheon last month, and she sat across the table from us. She had on that red hat that we both liked so much.

Annette: That's it! I remember the hat. Now I remember who Janet is. She recently moved into that new condo in our neighborhood. In fact, I remember liking her very much. Thanks for the help.

What happened was that Annette didn't make a connection to Janet's name, but she had a good connection to the red hat. By asking for more stimuli, you increase your probability of finding a connection you can use.

Follow-up: Practice each of these strategies the next time you are looking for that fact that is right on the tip of your tongue!

Schemata

In a letter to Robert Hooke,[3] Sir Isaac Newton wrote, "If I have seen further (than you and Descartes) it is by standing upon the shoulders of Giants."

Sir Isaac was referring to great scientists who had made so many contributions before him and from whom he had learned so very much that he did not have to *rediscover* their facts to advance science in the way that he did. This notion is the essence of *schemata*. New ideas rarely exist in a complete vacuum. They are related to other experiences, and we can borrow the knowledge from those experiences to learn new information.

For example, think about filling your car with gasoline. You know the general plan for accomplishing that task. When you arrive at a new gas station, or when your regular station gets reconfigured with new pumps, you do not have to learn completely from the beginning how to pump the gas into your car. You know the general scheme of pumping gas. You need only to learn what is different from what you already know. Use schemas to help you retrieve memories by asking yourself, "How is the problem at hand similar to something I already know?"

The strategies that use schemata include asking yourself two questions:

1. What is the same that I already know?
2. What is different from what I already know?

He said, she said.

In this exercise, you will practice schema theory by identifying the topic of these cryptic conversations. Check your answers at the end of this chapter in "Solutions to Exercises and Games."

The Call

He said: Did you call?

She said: Yes.

He said: How long?

She said: They promised to deliver within 25 minutes.

He said: What toppings?

She said: The usual.

What are they talking about? _____

Two, Please

He said: Two, please.

She said: $11.50.

He said: Here you go. What time does it start?

She said: 7:35. Second door on the left. Thank you.

Where are they? _____

How's That?

He said: How's that feel?

She said: Good. Do you have it in blue?

He said: Yes, ma'am.

She said: Mmh, too tight. Does it come in a narrow?

He said: I think it does. Excuse me for a minute.

What is happening? _____

Follow-up: Create *he said, she said* conversations of your own and ask another person what the conversation is about.

Compare and Contrast

In each of the following pictures, determine how the objects are alike. Then identify a distinguishing characteristic that discriminates the object on the right from the other objects in the group. Check your answers at the end of this chapter in "Solutions to Exercises and Games."

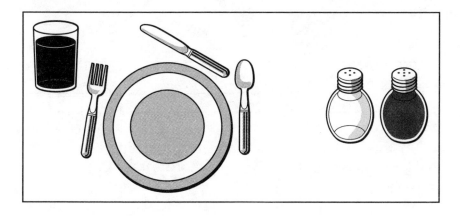

Figure 4-6: _____

_____

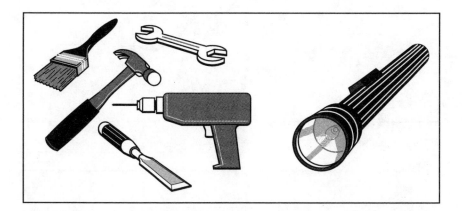

Figure 4-7: _____

_____

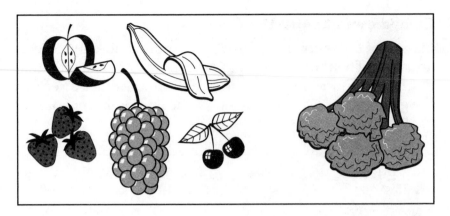

Figure 4-8: _____

_____

In this figure, find as many relationships as you can. Look for groups of two, three, or more items.

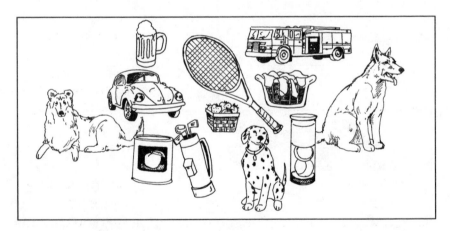

Figure 4-9: _____

_____

Follow-up: In each group of objects you encounter, look for common characteristics as well as distinguishing characteristics of its members.

Time Allowed to Search

Harmeyer's Law of Problem Solving states that 95 percent of your ability to solve a problem rests entirely in two beliefs:

1. A solution to the problem exists.
2. You can find the solution.

If either of these beliefs is compromised, you stop looking for the solution. The key to retrieving information is to keep looking for it. Allow yourself plenty of time to remember. Don't get frustrated with yourself if you cannot remember a fact in a split-second. The frustration will interfere with your search. Work through the search strategies you learned in this section.

Associations

The creation of *associations* refers to tying new information to already-learned information. Just as associations are formed by groups of people joined by a common interest, we can use common ideas to assist us in storing information in memory. You can make links or connections between what you want to learn and what you previously committed to memory. Thinking of one idea will cause you to think of the other. You can use this technique in all learning situations. The more associations you create, the more likely you will be able to recall the information successfully. This process is related to the expression *Don't put all your eggs in one basket*. If you have used several techniques to try to retain some information, you are in effect carrying your information in more than one basket. And if something happens to one basket, you can still access the eggs (information) in the other baskets.

One example is learning someone's name. Suppose that you encounter a woman named Janet. You might try to find something distinctive about her that reminds you of a planet to help you remember by a rhyming link. Perhaps she has a round face. When you see her face, it will remind you of a planet. Many names suit a person, and it is easy, once you get

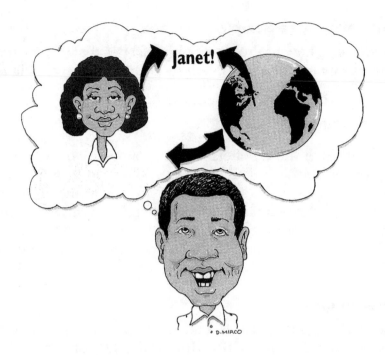

in the practice of it, to notice a link to a name. The name might be the name of a relative or another friend. It may not be wise to link a name to a garment, unless it is a uniform that person will be wearing at your next meeting.

Let's take another look at a scenario we discussed in Chapter 1. Do you remember the wife who used auditory, visual, and kinesthetic strategies and never forgot anything? Her strategies are much more robust than we implied and deserve a second look. She repeats to herself the thing she is trying to remember to do in an interesting rhyme or pattern *(verbal rehearsal, repetition priming, and coding)*, writes it down on a piece of paper, and puts it next to her place mat where she will see it as she eats her meals *(imagery, repetition priming)*; then she tells her husband to remind her *(repetition priming)*. She knows her husband will never remind her, and he knows she doesn't really expect him to remind her (so he doesn't bother to store it). They are operating on an accepted *schema pattern* here, where the circumstances of her telling him a fact are a memorable pattern. All the techniques combined create many associations between the information she needs to learn and the information she already has stored in her mind. Now you can truly understand why she never forgets a thing. You might try combining these or other techniques to see how well your ability to retain and recall information improves.

When You Say . . . I Say . . .

The associations you develop are going to be very personal. However, here is a little quiz that can help you appreciate the power of associations. You'll find some possible answers for these associations at the end of this chapter in "Solutions to Exercises and Games."

   1. When you say *salt*, I say _____.

   2. When you say *husband*, I say _____.

   3. When you say *Romeo*, I say _____.

   4. When you say *Abbott*, I say _____.

   5. When you say *Kitty Hawk*, I say _____.

   6. When you say *socks*, I say _____.

   7. When you say *north*, I say _____.

   8. When you say *up*, I say _____.

   9. When you say *January 15th*, I say _____.

 10. When you say *1776*, I say _____.

 11. When you say *Boise*, I say _____.

 12. When you say *needle*, I say _____.

Deck Four

You also can use associations as a storage technique. In this exercise, you will practice looking for connections by making associations and chunking information. Noticing connections is a skill rather than a talent, and developing this skill requires practice. Fortunately, there is an easy, low-cost method for looking for connections. You will need a deck of cards. Any set will do. This example uses a bridge deck.

Here's how: Deal four cards face up. Study the four cards and look for connections among the cards. Write down the connections you notice. Deal the next four cards, and continue until the deck is finished. Here are some connections to get your brain thinking in this direction:

- Look for the same number of pips on the cards—two of a kind, three of a kind, four of a kind. (*Pips* are spots on each card.)
- Look for a sequence of numbers—3, 4, 5 or 4, 6, 8.
- Look for all even or all odd numbers of pips on the cards.
- Try to sum two or three of the cards to equal the number of pips on the third or fourth card.
- Look for a birth date— 10♦ 3♣ 4♠ 5♥ might represent October 3, 1945.

Soon you will be noticing connections of your own. A sample run of a deck follows. Study our findings and look for connections in the last seven sets of cards. Check your answers at the end of this chapter in "Solutions to Exercises and Games."

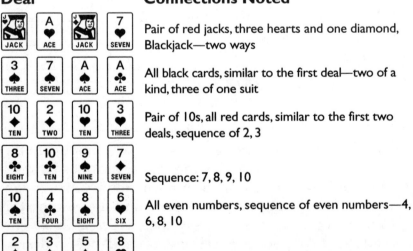

Deal	Connections Noted
J♥ A♥ J♦ 7♥	Pair of red jacks, three hearts and one diamond, Blackjack—two ways
3♠ 7♠ A♠ A♣	All black cards, similar to the first deal—two of a kind, three of one suit
10♦ 2♦ 10♥ 3♥	Pair of 10s, all red cards, similar to the first two deals, sequence of 2, 3
8♣ 10♣ 9♠ 7♦	Sequence: 7, 8, 9, 10
10♠ 4♣ 8♠ 6♥	All even numbers, sequence of even numbers—4, 6, 8, 10
2♠ 3♦ 5♦ 8♥	2 + 3 = 5; 3 + 5 = 8

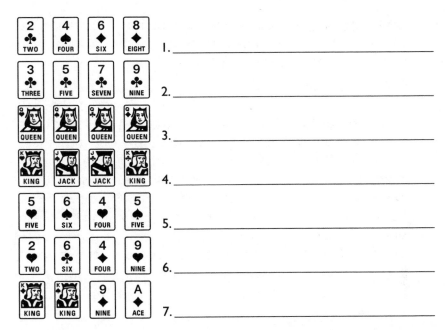

1._____

2._____

3._____

4._____

5._____

6._____

7._____

Follow-up: Find a deck of cards and deal again. Look at each of the four cards and try to find a connection within each set of four cards.

If you are outdoors, you can play this game with license plates. Find a connection among the digits on the plate. Do the same for the letters. Look for all stick letters (A, V, M), rounded letters (O, C, S), and combination stick and curve (P, D, B). Be creative! But don't let it interfere with your driving!

PREPARING FOR YOUR INFORMATION-PROCESSING POSTASSESSMENT

Before you do your postassessment, let's see how you might apply some of the techniques of this chapter to the information-processing preassessment. First, refresh your mind by rereading the shopping scenario on page 83.

Here are some examples of how you might have used the information-processing techniques of this chapter to help you remember the items on your errands list:

- **Imaging:** Look for the list in your memory. Visualize the place where you wrote the items on the list. You may be able to see the paper in your mind. If so, read it!

- **Coding:** If you encode the list of the items before you leave the house, you might be able to recall the list. How about using your body as the code? Start at the top with your head. Your hair is on top—get your sister at the beauty shop. Next your mouth: You need to get a prescription as well as the groceries. Then your clothes, watch, and shoes are on your body. You need your hands to buy birthday cards. In your purse or pockets, you carry money, so go to the bank. Keep scanning over your body until you have accomplished all the tasks.

- **Mnemonics:** Try to find a phrase to remind you of the stops: cleaners, shoe repair, druggist, watch repair, grocery, beauty shop, bank. You might want to rearrange the list to find a good mnemonic. We found this one: SGDBBCW—Some Great Danes bark, but collies wag.

- **Hierarchy:** You will need a device for the list of items at the grocery store. Use the food pyramid to organize the foods you need: sweets at the top (ice cream), then meat and dairy (soup), next fruits and vegetables (bananas), and bottom grains (breads and rice).

- **Associations:** There will be some help in the car with you. You will have the shirts and suit with you. That should remind you of the cleaners trip. Associate picking up with dropping off—that is, the shoes with the clothing.

- **Auditory learning-style preference:** Read the items aloud before leaving the house.

- **Visual learning-style preference:** Look over the list before you leave the house.

- **Kinesthetic learning-style preference:** See yourself at each of the stops before leaving the house.

- **Spatial:** Plan your route before you leave the house. Plan to take the shortest route to all of the stops. Number the stops on the list in the order you will make them. This planning session alone will rehearse the list of errands in meaningful arrangements. Your brain will take notice that this is important information, and perhaps some of it will linger in short-term memory long enough for you to accomplish your tasks.

Notice that we did not explicitly remember the list of items at the cleaners. They probably will not require a list. You most likely have the ticket for the cleaners, and if not, the cleaners has a record of what you dropped off. Spend your time and mental energy on the items for which you do not have a ready prompt.

INFORMATION-PROCESSING POSTASSESSMENT

Keep these various learning strategies in mind as you study the next few paragraphs. For example, make associations, develop mnemonics, look for hierarchies, and use repetition.

You are going out to finish the last of your holiday shopping. You need to be sure that your uncle Lewis, your spouse's cousin Edward, and niece Shara each have two gifts. The two gifts should total no more than $30. Lewis has just bought a new Chevy truck. Edward is environmentally conscious, and Shara is bubbly and energetic.

You already have bought several gifts during off-season sales, with the intention of deciding who gets what later, and have them stored in your closet at home. The items and their values are

Aluminum-can crusher	$10
Interstate highway map	$15
Recycling bins	$20

You decide to give Edward the can crusher as well as the recycling bins and to give Lewis the map.

You drive to the local mall with the intention of visiting several stores, getting a quick bite for lunch, checking with several other stores if you have not found what you are looking for, and then returning home. At the mall, you go first to the department store, where you find a lovely perfume named *Happy* and decide to buy that for your niece. It costs $25 dollars a bottle. Next, you visit a clothing store, where you find a bright yellow shirt that would be just perfect for Shara marked down to $5 (a wonderful bargain). You look through two gift shops but find nothing appropriate. Tired but running late, you grab a soft drink and keep looking.

The next two shops, a men's clothing store and a sporting goods store, do not have any suitable items. But at the end of the mall is a recreation vehicle specialty store, and you find a travel mug priced at $7, which you purchase for your uncle. Relieved you have completed your shopping, you return home. Turn to page 120 to answer the questions.

(continue to the next page)

Questions

1. What is your uncle's name? _____

2. What is your price limit on the two gifts? _____

3. What items did you already have at home?_____

4. What is the name of the perfume you bought your niece? _____

5. Where did you have lunch? _____

6. What gifts are you giving to your uncle?_____
   _____

7. What did you find at the sporting goods store? _____
   _____

8. What did you buy for Edward? _____
   _____

9. What was your great bargain? _____
   _____

10. Is Edward your cousin? _____

Check your answers in "Solutions to Exercises and Games." Compare your results with those of your preassessment.

- Did you improve over the information-processing pre-assessment?
- How did your scores compare?
- How many of the new techniques did you employ?

The more of these techniques you can use, the better your performance will be on problems like this.

 Continue to practice these techniques. Find a way to practice one technique each day. Check our Web site daily (www.mentalagility.com) to see what helpful hint we can give you that day regarding a learning technique or strategy.

This chapter, believe it or not, has just touched the tip of the iceberg (visual imagery) regarding the use of information-processing strategies in your everyday life. We are going to take a brief expedition in Chapter 5, "Support the Aging Brain," to discover the effects of aging on our systems so that we can combine compensation and accommodation strategies with our information-processing techniques. Chapters 6, "Regain an Agile Brain," and 7, "Enjoy Your Ageless Mental Agility," will present a more robust treatment of the ideas found in Chapters 4 and 5 and will introduce new, more advanced techniques.

SOLUTIONS TO EXERCISES AND GAMES

Information-Processing Preassessment

Solution: Give yourself one point for each of the following answers:

1. bread, ice cream, bananas, rice, and soup
2. my sister
3. no
4. Ruth
5. six shirts and a suit
6. watch repair, drugstore, shoe repair, and bank
7. the bank
8. Nothing—the hardware store is not on my list of errands.
9. No, I need to *pick up* the shoes.
10. Two birthday cards and a prescription.

The Advantages of Repetition Priming

Solutions: 1. Ivory soap **2.** Ajax **3.** Preference hair color **4.** Nike sports equipment **5.** Roto-Rooter **6.** NBC television network **7.** Campbell's soup **8.** Hellman's mayonnaise **9.** United Airlines **10.** Hallmark cards **11.** Kentucky Fried Chicken (KFC) **12.** Exxon gasoline **13.** Wheaties cereal **14.** Frosted Flakes cereal **15.** Baskin Robbins

Imagine That

Solutions: You may have different experiences and therefore richer answers than those listed here. **1.** the bottom right **2.** above the nose **3.** This varies—three or four tines are common. **4.** lowercase **5.** clockwise **6.** depends on which side of the door the lock is **7.** counterclockwise **8.** halfway between the 7 and the 8 **9.** counterclockwise **10.** left side **11.** away from the doorjamb **12.** two **13.** on the right side **14.** ℞ **15.** Across the top of the alphabetic keys. Additionally, some computer keyboards have a numeric keypad at the right of the keyboard. **16.** bottom row **17.** top row **18.** top row **19.** C **20.** S

Demonic Mnemonics

Solutions: 1. f **2.** h **3.** d (Hint: Count the number of letters in each of the words in the prompt. **4.** a **5.** i **6.** e **7.** c **8.** g **9.** j **10.** b

If It Looks Like a Duck and Walks Like a Duck . . .

Solutions: You may have identified different classes. This is merely a list of possible answers. **1.** kinds of dogs **2.** kinds of dishes **3.** kinds of children's pets **4.** things that start with "a" **5.** words that contain double vowels **6.** cities that are state capitals **7.** things that are roots **8.** things that are spelled the same backward and forward (palindromes) **9.** things that are spelled with five letters **10.** things that have wings **11.** things you can play **12.** things you can read **13.** things that have falls **14.** things that run **15.** things that have seals

He Said, She Said

Solutions: The call: They are talking about pizza. **Two, please:** They are at the movies. **How's that?:** They are in a shoe store.

Compare and Contrast

Solutions: You may have noticed different similarities and differences. This is a sample of what we noticed. **Figure 4-6:**

All the items belong on the dinner table. Exclusively one diner uses the objects on the left. The salt and pepper may be used by all of the diners. **Figure 4-7:** All the objects are tools. The flashlight is the only one that requires batteries and the only one that is not mechanical. **Figure 4-8:** All the objects are food. All items on the left are fruit, and the broccoli is a vegetable. **Figure 4-9:** Answers may vary with each reader's creativity and the many relationships among the objects drawn. Some examples are things in cans, things for sports, dogs, things from Germany.

When You Say . . . I Say . . .

Solutions: You may have different associations for these prompts. These are sample responses. **1.** pepper **2.** wife **3.** Juliet **4.** Costello **5.** the Wright brothers **6.** shoes (or the Clintons' cat) **7.** south **8.** down **9.** Dr. Martin Luther King, Jr. **10.** Declaration of Independence **11.** Idaho **12.** thread, or perhaps haystack

Deck Four

Solutions: 1. all even numbers, in a sequence **2.** all odd numbers in a sequence **3.** all queens **4.** two pairs, Kings and Jacks; all of them are male cards **5.** $6 + 4 = 10$ and $5 + 5 = 10$ **6.** February 6, 1949 **7.** pair of Kings, each worth 10 points, and $9 + A$ counts at 10 points as well

Information-Processing Postassessment

A good attack on this problem is to make an association for person-relation-interest-gift-gift. That will help you figure out most of the answers.

Solutions: Give yourself one point for each of the following answers:

1. Lewis

2. $30

3. aluminum-can crusher, interstate highway map, and recycling bins

4. Happy

5. I didn't have lunch; I grabbed a soft drink.

6. travel mug and interstate highway map

7. nothing

8. You bought nothing on this trip. However, on previous trips, you bought the aluminum-can crusher and recycling bins. Give yourself credit for either answer.

9. the bright yellow shirt

10. No, he is my spouse's cousin.

REFERENCES:

1. L.L. Jacoby and M. Dallas, "On the Relationship between Autobiographical Memory and Perceptual Learning, " *Journal of Experimental Psychology: General 110* (1981): 306–340.

2. David Sousa, Ph.D., *How the Brain Learns* (NASSP, 1995)

3. *Bartlett's Familiar Quotations* (Brown and Company, Inc., 1980).

C h a p t e r

5

Support the Aging Brain

Orchestrate the Interplay Between Mind and Body

KEY CONCEPTS

Physical Aspects of Aging
Psychological Aspects of Aging
Cognitive Aspects of Aging

INTRODUCTION

"Youth is a disease from which we all recover." — **Dorothy Fuldheim**

FACTS ABOUT AGING QUIZ

Test your knowledge about the aging process with these 12 statements about aging. Read each one and determine whether it is true or false.

1. _____ As people age, they experience reduced muscle strength.

2. _____ Oral health declines as a result of the aging process.

3. _____ Approximately 25 percent of all older adults develop corneal cataracts.

4. _____ It is normal to become more forgetful as you age.

5. _____ According to the National Institute of Aging, 85 percent of all those over 85 years old live in residential communities or nursing homes.

6. _____ Senility is inevitable in older people.

7. _____ Women's sexual desire declines sharply as they age.

8. _____ Incontinence is a normal part of aging.

9. _____ Elders should prepare themselves and their families for their deaths by withdrawing from family activities.

10. _____ The effects of prescription drugs diminish as we age, so larger doses are required to gain the same effects as before.

11. _____ Seniors experience less stress because of their relaxed lifestyle.

12. _____ 75 percent of seniors dread getting older.

All the statements in the quiz you just took are false. They are all common misconceptions of the aging process.

The changes in our physical and mental abilities presented in this chapter are generalizations. The exact amount of the change is not the same for each individual. For example, you know individuals whose hearing has declined (some more than others) and other individuals whose hearing remains unchanged. So when you read research results or articles in newspapers that say "this" happens as we age, remember that "this" is not written in stone. "This" depends on individual characteristics, such as health and lifestyles and may be true for some and not for others.

Speaking of research results, it is important to you as a consumer of information to understand the manner in which experimental results regarding the effects of aging are obtained. Many research projects are cross sectional in format. That means the comparisons are between, let's say, a group of

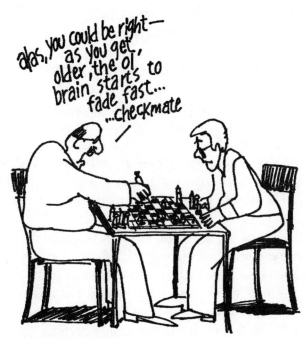

Reprinted with permission.

20-year-olds and a different group of 70-year-olds. In some ways, this is like comparing apples to oranges. You don't know what educational, economic, or environmental background the participants experienced as they reached their present age. Their health and lifestyles may be quite diverse. The relevance of such tests sometimes is questionable when discussing the effects of age on cognitive and physical functions of individuals. However, a *longitudinal study,* in which specific individuals are tested as they progress in age, yields a true comparison of aging effects on an individual. Not as many longitudinal studies are performed as cross-sectional studies because of the expense and difficulties involved in tracking and evaluating people through many years.

Another problem with many of the tests administered is the lack of connection of the tests to real life. Many tests are abstract in nature. Seeing how many numbers you can memorize, how quickly you can turn a lever, and so on are not relevant to a senior's life. Some experts believe that the

seniors do not compete or try as hard as the younger participants, who may have participated more recently in test situations in school.

Many studies concentrate on anticipated declines of abilities. Researchers feel the need to find declining abilities to try
to prevent or minimize these declines. "Information about
cognitive abilities that remain stable or increase with age, although perhaps desirable to provide a more balanced por-
trayal of the true capabilities of older adults, has a lower
priority among many researchers because it has been pre-
sumed to be of less value in contributing to the ultimate elim-
ination of age-related cognitive problems."[1]

Thus, many of the results of aging that have been published are disheartening, to say the least. However, retirement
also would be distressing if we were not fully prepared with
compensation strategies (part-time jobs and mortgage pre-
payment to stretch our dollars) and accommodations (volunteer work and travel to fill free time). So let's take a hard look
at aging's effect on our bodies and minds. Then you can begin
to prepare compensation and accommodation strategies to
have enjoyable and successful senior years.

Retirement is an accepted, normal part of aging, and if
prepared for properly, a time of life we cheerfully anticipate.
We prepare for retirement by evaluating present circumstances and anticipating future changes in our economic situation. Some individuals start earlier preparations, use
better strategies, and thus are more prepared than others.

Just as we want to be one of the more successful design-
ers of our economic future, we want to be one of the more effective analyzers of our physical and mental supply and
demand. It is critical to our successful aging to be aware of
potential changes in our bodies and mental supply and demand. You must prepare to maximize the good and minimize the bad effects of the aging process.

> *"Old age is like everything else. To make a success of
> it you have to start young." — Fred Astaire*

The younger you are when you begin to plan for aging, the healthier and more active you will be mentally and physically for more years. However, as the old saying goes, *Better later than never.* Don't wait until tomorrow or next week to start. Determine today that you are going to take charge of how you age and not just accept whatever happens to you. Only 35 percent of how you age is determined by genetics; the rest is determined by your lifestyle, environment, and other factors—many of which you can control and alter.

PHYSICAL ASPECTS OF AGING

As we age, our sensations and perceptions, our "bridges" to the world, may change and begin to decline. Some of our abilities to interact with and interpret the world correctly then may be dependent on our ability to perceive the world accurately and efficiently. As a matter of fact, some researchers believe that most of the declines traditionally attributed to senior's cognitive abilities are actually the result of inaccuracies in obtaining and processing information through our five senses.[2] The following discussion describes each of the five senses, our physical support structure, sleep requirements, and reaction times as they affect our mental abilities.

Vision

The single most important thing you can do for your eyesight is to get an eye exam every one to two years. If you are a visual learner, sight is your primary mechanism for gathering information. Inaccuracies in judgments may be the result of erroneously perceived information. It is imperative that you have regular eye exams. Not only do you need someone to prescribe the proper corrective lenses, but early detection of diseases such as glaucoma and macular degeneration is essential to reduce damage.

A profound loss of vision is not normal.

The lens of the eye begins to stiffen in middle childhood, and we begin to focus less precisely. The decline is gradual and may not be noticed until the mid-thirties or mid-forties. For some people, this condition is corrected by glasses, contact lenses, or laser surgery. For declines in near- and far-sighted vision, glasses or contacts are compensation mechanisms. If you have progressed to bifocal prescriptions, you might consider *monovision*. This is a technique where a person wears two different lenses, one for nearsightedness and one for farsightedness. It takes most people approximately seven to 10 days to adjust, although a few people never adjust. If an eye exam reveals that you need a simple pair of reading glasses, you can get them at a drugstore. Just be sure that you get a professional exam, instead of self-prescribing, so that you can be checked for conditions such as glaucoma.

Other changes in vision can be attributed to diseases such as glaucoma, cataracts, or macular degeneration. Regular eye examinations allow for early detection that can stop or slow disease progression. *Glaucoma* damages peripheral vision first and then moves on to destroy central vision. Glaucoma is the result of pressure on the optic nerve. Medicated eyedrops have been the most popular and prevalent treatment, but recently laser surgery has been successful as a treatment. Glaucoma sometimes is referred to as a *silent blinder.* By the time you realize that something is wrong, the disease has progressed to an advanced stage. If you have a family history of glaucoma, are African-American, or are diabetic, your chances of developing glaucoma are higher than normal, and you should be especially conscientious about scheduling yearly eye exams.

Macular degeneration affects the central part of the retina, which allows you to see details. Peripheral vision remains intact. Some of the symptoms are dark spots in the center of the vision area, blurring, and line distortion. Eye specialists often recommend special vitamins to combat this disease. Dark green leafy vegetables are high in carotenoids and reduce the risk of advanced macular degeneration by 43 percent.[3]

Remember that the best foods for us are the most brightly colored ones.

Cataracts, another physical condition common to the aging of our eyes, are a clouding of the lens. In fact, some say that cataracts are inevitable, but we know some 90-year-olds who don't appear to have cataracts. Of course, they may just be aging at a different rate and they don't show yet. The symptoms of a cataract are double vision in one eye, colors appear less bright, and decreased light sensitivity. The good news is that cataracts are corrected easily by surgery.

It is also thought that reducing the eye's exposure to ultraviolet light reduces damage to the lens. You should wear sunglasses that are labeled indicating that they block 99 percent of both Ultraviolet A and Ultraviolet B light. Wearing a broad-brimmed hat while outdoors also reduces the amount of ultraviolet light to which the eye is exposed.

One of the changes in our perceptions that research has identified is that our perceptual window narrows. We do not scan a large area as easily as when we were younger and need to break a large visual area into smaller sections to identify a target object. In other words, if we took our family for an outing and stood looking at a picturesque street scene, the younger members might take it all in at a glance. Older members of the family might subconsciously break the street into sections and look each one over for details. We need to focus on smaller sections of the environment.

Upon occasion, I have "lost" my car in the parking lot. So, while I try to look like I know where I am going, I begin to scan the parking lot looking for my blue car among all the other cars. I don't have to slow down the scanning process and check out the nonblue cars as I come across them. However, the blue cars are all potentially mine, and I have to slow down and look more carefully to determine whether it is my blue car. To increase my speed and accuracy, I need to break the parking lot into sections and quickly scan one section at a time instead of looking repeatedly over the entire parking lot. Of course, if you have a general idea of where your car is located, you can just scan that one area. The simplest thing, I suppose, would be to tie something bright to the radio antenna and look for that. I think I'll do that!

We also become fractions of a second slower at identifying specific targets in a cluttered environment. A few hundredths of a second may not be important, or even noticeable to others, when looking for your car in a parking lot. Nevertheless, this fraction-of-a-second delay could contribute to an accident if you are driving a car. If you are traveling in a car at 60 miles per hour (88 feet per second), a delay of just one-tenth second results in your car being almost nine feet farther along the road, possibly running into a stopped car in front of you. So get your eyes tested, take your vitamins, wear your glasses, and give yourself a little extra time to identify objects visually.

Hearing

A gradual loss of hearing sensitivity begins in young adulthood. After age 50, approximately 70 percent of the population has some form of hearing loss. Hearing loss may affect all sound frequencies or just specific frequencies. I have a friend named Shelly, for example, who is legally deaf. Shelly can hear the pitch of my voice and yet cannot understand what someone with a deep, booming, very loud voice says. It's not the loudness of the sound, it's the pitch that affects her hearing. Not all adults suffer from loss of hearing.

A profound loss of hearing is not normal.

It may help to have a working definition for the degrees of hearing impairment as we continue our discussion about hearing. This table gives you a simple measurement scale of the degree of hearing loss you or someone you know may experience.

If you	You may have
Can hear a whisper at 20 feet	No hearing loss
Cannot hear a whisper at 3 feet	Moderate hearing loss
Cannot hear a conversational voice 1 foot away	Severe hearing loss
Cannot hear a shout with someone's mouth next to your ear	Profound hearing loss

Men usually have more extensive and more rapid hearing loss than women. Women tend to retain their hearing ability. People who have had to work or live in areas that expose them to damaging noise levels experience a more significant loss of hearing as they age. City dwellers and industrial workers experience greater hearing loss than those living in rural settings because of the constant exposure to background noise.

This is the case with Kathleen's father, Glenn Austin, whose office was located on the shop floor of an aircraft production plant with a constant high-level noise environment.

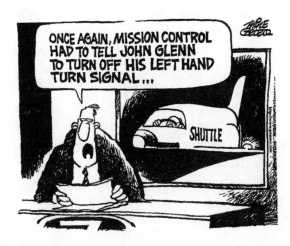

© Tribune Media Services, 1998. All Rights Reserved. Reprinted with permission.

However, his problem is just the opposite of Shelly's: it's with high-frequency sounds. His daughters deliberately try to lower the pitch of their voices when they speak to him.

Certain medications, such as those that reduce high blood pressure and inflammation, can decrease hearing effectiveness in the high-frequency range.[4] You must have your hearing checked. Just because you hear some sound frequencies does not mean that you are hearing all sound frequencies at a safe level.

This loss of hearing may have a great impact on social interaction. Asking people to repeat their conversations may cause older adults to become embarrassed, frustrated, and avoid interactions with others. You can use many strategies to accommodate this decline, however. An undesirable strategy is to pretend that you know what the person said. The consequences of this are not very appealing. Some people with hearing loss try to "listen in context." This means that if they miss a word or two, they continue listening to deduce what the speaker *may* have said. At times this is a useful strategy, but the consequences might be dreadful if the deduction is incorrect!

For those who sustain gradual hearing loss, there is a natural tendency to make accommodations. This anecdote is an example of how one senior citizen made an accommodation for his hearing loss. When someone spoke to him and he heard something, but not clearly and completely, he tried to determine from the portion he did hear and the circumstances involved what must have been said. At first, he found this to be a dangerous practice. He may nod "yes" in the wrong places. Noting the reaction to your response becomes very important. Soon he became very adept at observing nonverbal reactions. It became automatic—like a minicomputer was doing it. After a while, he agreed that he needed a hearing aid. When he was being tested, an audiologist assumed he must be lip reading, because he was responding to questions so well without a hearing aid, despite a significant hearing loss. When the elder said he didn't know how to lip read, the audiologist blindfolded him to check this out. The elder still was able to respond appropriately. The audiologist concluded that the elder was "listening in context" and not lip reading. This would seem to be a natural accommodation and probably not unique.

More positive compensation strategies include the following actions. You can eliminate competing sounds such as the TV or radio by turning them off. If a speaker talks too quickly, you can ask him to slow down or speak more clearly. You also might be able to rearrange your sitting area so that you can sit across from your visitors and more clearly see their mouths and faces to help you interpret their speech. Try these adjustments to boost your ability to carry on a conversation better. Stay in the conversation longer for more enjoyment!

When conversing with someone who may be using your nonverbal cues, give him time to do the processing. If the information you are passing on is critical, however, use the old tried-and-true formula: have him repeat the information back to you.

Hearing degradation can be dangerous—we use our hearing to warn us of many dangers. Is the heater running constantly? Is someone breaking in?

One of the simplest ways to minimize the effect of this decline is the use of a hearing aid. Amazingly, many people refuse to wear a hearing aid, even though the new hearing aids are very effective and fit into the ear canal so as to be invisible. In one research study, of those individuals who found it difficult to follow a conversation in a crowded room, 75 percent did not use a hearing aid. We have an aunt who always prefaces advice with "If you get cold, you get a sweater, if you get hungry, you get something to eat." She would be the first to say "If you can't hear, you might investigate getting a hearing aid."

A Five-Minute Hearing Test Especially for Seniors

This test is from the *American Academy of Otolaryngology– Head and Neck Surgery Public Service Brochure.* Answer each of the following questions by placing a checkmark in the column that is most like you. You'll find a scoring guide after the test.

Question	Almost Always	Half the time	On Occasion	Never
I have a problem hearing over the telephone.	_____	_____	_____	_____
I have trouble following the conversation when two or more people are talking at the same time.	_____	_____	_____	_____
People complain that I turn the TV volume up too high.	_____	_____	_____	_____
I have to strain to understand conversations.	_____	_____	_____	_____
I miss hearing some common sounds like the phone or doorbell ringing.	_____	_____	_____	_____
I have trouble hearing conversations in a noisy background such as a party.	_____	_____	_____	_____
I get confused about where sounds come from.	_____	_____	_____	_____
I misunderstand some words in a sentence and need to ask people to repeat themselves.	_____	_____	_____	_____
I especially have trouble understanding the speech of women and children.	_____	_____	_____	_____
I have worked in noisy environments (assembly line, jackhammers, jet engines, and so on).	_____	_____	_____	_____

Many people I talk to seem to mumble (or don't speak clearly).	_____	_____	_____	_____
People get annoyed because I misunderstand what they say.	_____	_____	_____	_____
I mis-understand what others are saying and make inappropriate responses.	_____	_____	_____	_____
I avoid social activities because I cannot hear well and fear I'll reply improperly.	_____	_____	_____	_____

To be answered by a family member or friend:

| Do you think this person has a hearing loss? | _____ | _____ | _____ | _____ |
| **Totals:** | _____ | _____ | _____ | _____ |

Scoring

To calculate your score, give yourself three points for every time you checked the Almost Always column, two for every Half the Time, one for every On Occasion, and 0 for every Never. If you have a blood relative who has a hearing loss, add another three points. Then total your points and find your score in the following table.

The American Academy of Otolaryngology–Head and Neck

Score	Surgery Recommendation
0–5	Your hearing is fine. No action is required.
6–9	Suggest you see an *ear nose and throat* (ENT) specialist.
10+	Strongly recommend you see an ENT specialist.

This quiz was field tested on 71 older patients in five cities; audiograms also were run on them. Results showed that those whose quiz scores indicated a need to see a physician were confirmed, on the audiogram, as having a hearing impairment.[5]

Taste

In general, the decrease in taste sensitivity with age is due to fewer taste buds, decreased salivary secretions, formation of fissures on the tongue, and age-related changes in the process of taste sensations by the central nervous system. This affects our quality and enjoyment of life. Nothing tastes right anymore. We do not enjoy eating and may decide it is not worth the trouble to cook or go out to eat. We may not get all the nutrition we need to feed our muscles, organs, and brains.

A profound loss of taste is not normal.

You might want to consider this as an opportunity to be adventurous and try new foods. How about the foods you tried before and did not like? Your tastes have changed, so perhaps you should give foods you did not like a second chance. Try hot sauce, anchovies, new fruits, and new vegetables. Use this opportunity to investigate new cooking styles. You might be careful when adding spices to your foods for company. They may find it a little strong!

Smell

olfactory—relating to the sense of smell

In general, some mild decrease of olfactory sensitivity is common with increasing age. Olfactory sensory receptor cells decrease in number as you age. A decrease in smell may influence our sensitivity to taste (as in when you have a cold). The smell of foods actually starts the digestive process because it triggers the release of insulin. This, in turn, influences our tastes, diet, and nutrition. In addition, a decrease in olfactory abilities could affect our safety if we cannot detect a gas leak or notice the smell of spoiled foods.

Some dentures have an effect on your sense of smell. Those dentures with a full upper plate across the roof of the mouth interfere with the absorption of the aroma of foods. If you have a set of these dentures and you notice that food does not smell or taste as well as before, consult with your dentist about the possibility of a different style with a partial upper plate.

A profound loss of smell is not normal.

Research at the University of Pennsylvania Medical Center's Smell and Taste Center indicates that a profound loss of smell is not normal and should be reported to your physician. Although many physicians do not ask about your sense of smell during an examination, a drastic loss of smell is one of the initial signs of neurodegenerative diseases, such as Alzheimer's, Parkinson's, multiple sclerosis, and others.[6] Keep in mind that if you have started a new medication, it might be the medication that suddenly has affected your sense of smell and taste. You might want to check with your physician and pharmacist about possible side effects of your medications.

> **neurodegenerative**—*relating to the decline of the powers of the brain*

Touch

Touch is a combination of sensitivities to pressure, pain, and heat/cold. Not a lot of information is available on the changes to these sensitivities as we age. There is evidence that our sensitivity to pressure decreases. Although studies have been performed to determine the effects of aging on our perception of pain, it is difficult to pinpoint the exact effect, because so much of our evaluation of the pain is psychological. It just seems that some of us tolerate pain better than others. There is no clear-cut understanding of the changes with respect to pain. As far as our sensitivity to temperature differences, you are well aware that your body adjusts to gradual changes in temperature. In the middle of winter, for example, 45-degree temperatures seem warm after weeks of temperatures in the 20s to 30s. In the summer, however, a 45-degree temperature would seem very cold after weeks of temperatures in the 80s. It takes approximately three days for our bodies to adjust to new temperatures. That is why when you go to another part of the country on vacation, it takes about three days for your body to adjust to the new temperature and humidity.

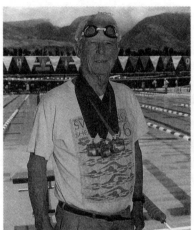

Photo courtesy of the Coon family

Older and Wiser

Dr. Jesse Coon is an excellent example of the benefits of exercising. A retired Texas A&M University professor, Jesse is 88 years old and an avid swimmer. He is in the 85- to 89-year-old age group of master swimmers, holds world records in the 50-meter and 100-meter butterfly, and holds national records in the 50-, 100-, and 200-yard butterfly and the 100- and 200-yard individual medley. Dr. Coon set these records in 1998, the year he turned 86, and they are still unbroken. He is looking forward to setting new records in the 90-and-older class.

Dr. Coon does not limit himself to swimming. He cross-trains with weights, is known as Captain Moonlighter in local sailing circles because of his devotion to sailing (and especially enjoys the moonlight excursions), and loves to dance. He is very active in his church and volunteers his time going to nursing homes and visiting with the patients.

Support Structure

Seniors suffer more than 1 million bone fractures annually. *Osteoporosis*, which means *porous bone*, is a condition of the bone in which the integrity of the bone structure is reduced, and breaks and fractures are more likely to occur. Many people believe it is a matter of clumsiness or carelessness that causes the senior to fall and break a bone.

Often the bone breaks first and then the senior falls.

The truth is that often seniors break a bone and *then* fall. This is due to loss of calcium in the bone structure. Although osteoporosis often is thought of as a woman's disease, half the patients being treated for osteoporosis are men. A simple, noninvasive bone-density test can determine your bone mass. In July 1998 Medicare began to pay for the bone-density test once each year.

To combat osteoporosis, weight-bearing activities such as walking and dancing cause bone cells to react by producing more bone cells and building stronger bones. Calcium supplements also help to reduce the loss of calcium and keep the bones strong. New prescription medicines approved by the *Food and Drug Administration* (FDA), such as FOSAMAX, help prevent bone loss. In addition, estrogen-replacement therapy for postmenopausal women (see Chapter 6 for more details) often is recommended to preserve bone tissue. Consult your physician concerning these and other therapies.

Muscles and the elastic cushioning of the vertebrae stiffen without proper exercises. Because 62 percent of those over the age of 65 do not exercise at all, it is not surprising that many seniors complain of muscle aches, pains, and stiffness of the joints. Think of all that exercise can do for you: increase suppleness, strengthen bones, improve your balance, and reverse weakness. Exercise benefits us mentally as well, but we'll save that for Chapter 6, "Regain an Agile Brain."

Sleep Patterns

As you age, you may lay awake longer before you drift off to sleep. If you get up at the same time every day, you begin to experience an accumulating "sleep debt." You feel more tired as the days go by. A decrease in overall sleep begins at age 30 for many men and 50 for many women. By the age of 65, most seniors rarely experience an unbroken night's sleep. Research indicates that people between the ages of 73 and 92 have an average of 21 awakenings during a given night. Men experience these awakenings more often than women until about age 70, when both men and women exhibit the same patterns of wakefulness.[7] Remember that sleep is essential to long-term memory formation as well as an overall sense of well-being. You must have complete cycles of sleep. Often, forgetfulness may be due to a lack of sleep instead of a decline in cognitive abilities. Chapter 6 details more information about the effects of sleep on learning.

Lack of sleep affects your intelligence, memory, and ability to concentrate.

There are many sleep strategies to help meet the daily demands on your memory. You may want to talk to your physician about the use of a sleeping aid such as melatonin or sleeping pills. Please be aware that supplements such as melatonin are controversial, and you should check with your physician before you begin to take over-the-counter remedies such as these. Exercising your body during the day not only strengthens you physically but also expends energy and makes you ready for sleep. You also might try relaxation exercises, yoga, or the good old glass of warm milk prior to retiring.

Reaction and Retrieval Time

Reaction time is the amount of time it takes for an individual to respond to a stimulus. Average reaction time increases with increasing age for seniors as a group. However, some individuals 70 years old or older may react more quickly than an individual 30-year-old. Your performance depends

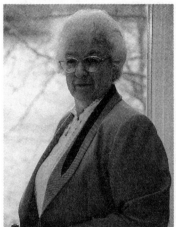

Photo courtesy of Winfield Leitzer

Older and Wiser

You couldn't find a busier person than Rita Gifford, 77, who is out and about volunteering her services, if not traveling around the world. Starting out as a den mother in the 1950s, she's been busy ever since. Rita has worked for her local historical society, raised funds for the Baltimore Symphony Orchestra, and given her time to visit a blind woman and take her to church. She and her husband, Bob, travel in the Elderhostels Education Program and have studied in Europe, Asia, and all over the USA—30 countries in all!

In 1980, Rita began a senior aerobics program. Her doctor thinks it may have saved her life. Early in 1994, Rita suffered the first of a series of life-threatening heart problems, ending with bypass surgery in 1996. One of the amazing things I notice about Rita is her unflappability. She persevered and did what was necessary to recover. Her positive attitude was a tremendous asset to her mending process.

And, yes, she's back at aerobics now that her doctor has given the go-ahead, and she is going strong!

on your mental agility and physical health, both of which you can improve.

It is possible that a 70-year-old person may take an average of up to one-fourth second longer to recognize an object in a picture than he did at the age of 30. Some researchers argue that this is a sign of cognitive decline. Many researchers, however, believe that this longer search and retrieval time might be due to the fact that the older we get, the more information we have stored, so it takes longer to search for the particular piece of information we need. After all, if you only have a few pieces of information in your "library" it doesn't take long to search through them all, but if you have thousands of facts and memories at you fingertips, it may indeed take you longer to find the relevant information. Isn't it uplifting to be thought of as a well-stocked library?

Adults also may be slower due to a lack of aerobic exercise. Aerobic exercises have been shown to improve individual reaction times. Because exercise increases blood flow to the brain, this suggests that longer reaction times may be caused by brain malnutrition. Physically active older people can have shorter reaction times than less-fit younger adults. So, with a little work and exercise, we have the potential to be better than we ever were!

Motivation may be important to reaction time and accuracy. Many older adults are just not interested in studies on speed. In one study, researchers shortened young and older adult reaction times and decreased the age difference in reaction time by making payment for participation partially contingent on speed of response.[8] In other words, make it relevant (or profitable), and older adults try harder and achieve more. Monetary reward is definitely a good incentive for trying harder.

PSYCHOLOGICAL ASPECTS OF AGING

There are those of us who relish getting older. The richness of life after 40 is wonderful, and over 50 is unbeatable. There are so many advantages to age—general knowledge, wisdom, self-knowledge, accomplishments, friends—that they are not readily countable. However, we live in a youth-centered culture where a common belief seems to be that the younger you are, the better. This is a notion obviously promoted by the young! At any rate, this tends to wear on us, and some older people actually believe that they would rather be young again.

"Age doesn't matter unless you are a cheese." — Billie Burke

Worrying about getting older actually hastens mental decline. We don't want you to worry about getting older. We want you to begin preparations for a superb aging process.

An old theory referred to disengagement of the senior adult as a necessary stage of life as you approached your last years. Removal from strenuous activity and interactions prepared the older adult to "pass on" and leave family members and friends behind. This theory was popular until the mid–1960s. Research has since demonstrated that the distancing of elders from others leads to physical and mental decline. Elders should not remove themselves from activities. They should recenter on what is important, stay engaged in interpersonal relationships, remain or become physically active, and maintain a stimulating mental environment.

Those who are happy and content with their lives show less cognitive decline than those suffering from stress or discontent.

Negative emotions, such as depression, anxiety, bitterness, and anger, cause mental abilities to decrease. Depression affects your motivation to remember, ability to concentrate, and perception of circumstances; it also causes overreactions to slight lapses in memory.[9] Moving can cause feelings of loneliness, grief, and an inability to concentrate. The reduction in responsibility and social contact after retirement may initially create feelings of a lack of purpose, sadness, and a sense of loss.

Staying active and engaged in life gives us reasons and opportunities to look forward to each day and to exercise those brain cells and practice remembering. Glenn Austin, 77, thinks that "there is no other lifestyle" than retirement!

COGNITIVE ASPECTS OF AGING

Several types of attention (concentration) abilities are compromised by age. We have trouble listening to two different things at once. If more than one person is trying to talk to us, we have trouble following either conversation. This may be due in part to a decrease in our hearing acuity. One of the conversationalists needs to wait.

We also have greater difficulty dividing our attention between two tasks. For example, we may experience greater difficulty trying to talk on the phone while hunting for an address in the phone book, or trying to talk to the cashier

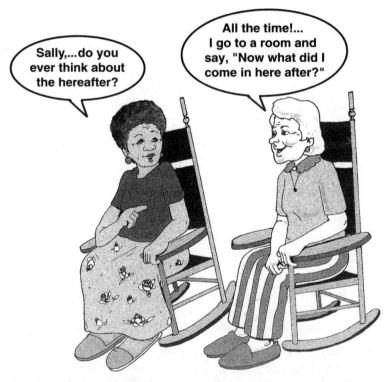

From Tal D. Bonham, *The Treasury of Clean Seniors' Jokes*, Nashville: Broadman and Holman Publishers, 1997, 72.

while we write a check. A failure in the ability to switch attention is evidenced when we go into the bedroom to look for a book and then cannot remember why we went in there. This problem is fairly common throughout life, and occurrences may increase as we age.

Much of the cognitive loss that is commonly considered a part of the aging process is actually attributable to extrinsic factors such as lack of practice, poor motivation, diet, health complications, and fatigue, and poor conditions of the testing, etc. The older we get, the more robust our store of information and knowledge becomes. We need to be more efficient at managing our mental resources. Actually, some researchers consider young people to be suffering from a handicap of inexperience and lack of wisdom for which they compensate with a speedy mind.[10]

Although it is commonly believed that age brings a loss of brain cells, new evidence points to neurogenesis—the birth of new neurons.

neurogenesis—the growth of new brain cells

Although it is true that the idle mind slows more rapidly than the lively mind, keeping it active is not enough. If you work a crossword puzzle every day, for example, you are exercising those particular areas of the brain each day. Those connections are strengthened and maintained. However, you want to stimulate other areas of the brain as well. Do you remember Figure 4-1, which compares the brain activity while learning a new task with brain activity after the task is more commonplace? If not, go peek again for another rehearsal. When stimulation is new and novel, other areas are incorporated into the thinking process. Your mind must be exposed to new experiences and stimuli to keep it agile. New stimuli cause new connections to be made, and blood flow to those areas increases within days. Nevertheless, as soon as the new activity becomes more or less routine, activity decreases.

You may have heard about the concept of lifelong learning. You definitely need to continue learning throughout life in order to stay mentally alert. This learning can take place in or out of a formal classroom setting. Just continue learning and exploring opportunities that you encounter in your life every day. If there is something that you always wanted to learn more about or learn how to do, this is a great opportunity to begin. Not only will it give you great pleasure and enjoyment, but it will keep those neurons in shape and increase the number of those connections.

Wisdom

Wisdom is expert knowledge about the fundamental issues of life. Wisdom has experience as the basis of sound judgment. As we age, we acquire insights into life's structure based on hindsight. Having solved many problems in our lives, we are good problem solvers. Seniors are more flexible, more comfortable with the ambiguities of life, and more context sensitive when applying problem-solving strategies to real-life situations. When faced with real-life problems, older subjects score consistently higher than younger subjects, trained therapists, and professional counselors.[11] As another example, although seniors read more slowly than the younger subjects, it was found that the seniors generated more ideas in general and more ideas central to the reading when asked to summarize. Many studies indicate that older adults compensate for slowing down by being more efficient at their tasks; although they may take a frac-

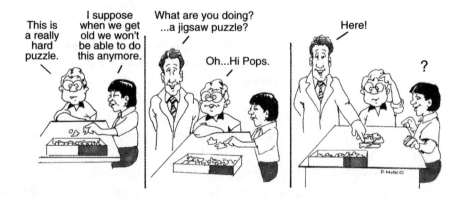

tion of a second longer to reach a decision, it is usually a better decision. Wisdom comes with age.

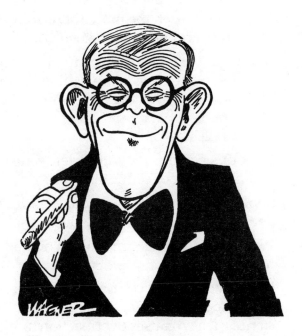

"You can't help getting older, but you don't have to get old."— George Burns

SELF-QUIZ

Test your new knowledge about the aging process with these 10 statements about aging. Read each one and determine whether it is true or false.

1. _____ Studies show that there may not be a decline in cognitive abilities in active, stimulated individuals. Intelligence test scores for these individuals may actually improve.

2. _____ People who are happy and content with their lives show less cognitive decline than those suffering from stress or discontent.

3. _____ The older we get, the more robust our store of information and knowledge becomes.

4. _____ Many people believe it is a matter of clumsiness, carelessness, or loss of coordination that causes seniors to fall and break a bone. Often the senior's bone breaks first, however, and then the senior falls.

5. _____ Lack of sleep affects your intelligence, memory, and ability to concentrate.

6. _____ Some individuals 70 years old or older may have better reaction times than a 30-year-old.

7. _____ Worrying about getting older actually hastens mental decline.

8. _____ Depression affects your motivation to remember, ability to concentrate, and perception of circumstances; it also causes overreaction to slight lapses in memory.

9. _____ Much of the cognitive loss that is commonly considered a part of the aging process is actually attributable to extrinsic factors such as lack of practice, poor motivation, diet, health complications, fatigue, and poor conditions of the testing.

10. _____ The best foods for us are the most brightly colored ones.

Some studies show that there may not be a decline in cognitive abilities in active, stimulated individuals. Intelligence test scores for mentally active individuals may actually improve. For those individuals whose mental skills have begun to decline, K. Warner Schaie's Seattle Longitudinal Study showed that, with practice, they could score as well as they had 14 years before. Moreover, this increased mental agility could be maintained for years.[12] Chapters 6,

"Regain an Agile Brain," and 7, "Enjoy Your Ageless Mental Agility," address these issues and provide you with many, many suggestions and activities to improve your mental acuity. You will learn and practice specific and detailed strategies to increase your education, keep you physically fit, increase your self-esteem, and keep you mentally fit. The younger you are when you begin to apply these strategies, the better off you will be.[13]

And by the way, all the statements on the quiz you just took are true. They are all results of recent research into the aging process.

REFERENCES:

1. Timothy Salthouse, *Theoretical Perspectives on Cognitive Aging* (New York: Lawrenece Erlbaum, 1991).
2. U. Lindenberger and P. B. Baltes, "Sensory functioning and intelligence in old age: A strong connection," *Psychology and Aging 9* (1994): 339–355
3. Martha Miller, "Your aging eyes," Better Homes and Gardens (July 1996): 46–51
4. *The 1998 Health Guide,* Baltimore County Department of Aging (Baltimore, Maryland, 1998).
5. The American Academy of Otolaryngology–Head and Neck Surgery, Inc., One Prince St., Alexandria VA 22314–3357, 1993.
6. Nancy Walsh D' Epiro, "Age and olfaction: An important warning sign," *Patient Care* (May 15, 1998): 14–15.
7. John J. Medina, *The Clock of Ages. Why we age – how we age – winding back the clock* (New York: Cambridge University Press, 1996).
8. A. Baron and W.R. Mattila, "Response slowing of older adults: Effects of time-limit contingencies on single- and dual-task performances," *Psychology and Aging 4* (1989): 66–72.
9. Alicia Di Rado, "UC Irvine Neuroscientists Tie Stress to Memory Lapses," *Nature* (August 19, 1998).

10. Joannie M. Schrof, "Brain Power," *U.S. News and World Report* (November 28, 1994): 89–97.
11. Fredda Blanchard-Fields, "The Role of Emotion in Social Cognition Across the Adult Life Span," *Annual Review of Gerontology and Geriatrics* 17 (1997). K. Warner Schaie and
M. Powell Lawton, eds. (New York: Springer Publishing Company).
12. K. Warner Schaie, *Intellectual Development in Adulthood* (Cambridge University Press, 1996).
13. John W. Rowe and Robert L. Kahn, *Successful Aging* (New York: Random House, 1998).

Chapter
6

Regain an Agile Brain

Implement Personalized Techniques to Redesign Your Aging Process

KEY CONCEPTS

Research Results
Rhythms of Your Brain
Resting Your Brain
Feeding Your Brain
Exercising Your Brain
Feeling with Your Brain
Protecting Your Brain

INTRODUCTION

Wouldn't it be wonderful if we could somehow slow the aging process, grow mentally younger, or amazingly, even regain our previous mental capabilities? Be able to think clearly and not experience the frustration of failing to recall an important piece of information? Former President George Bush had a suggestion:

> "I have long thought that the aging process could be slowed down, if it had to work its way through Congress."—George Bush

Well, perhaps Congress is not a very practical method to counteract the aging process. We need personal techniques that we can implement ourselves to control and combat the aging process. In Chapter 5, you read about the challenges to the aging brain. This chapter expands on proven methods and strategies you easily can integrate into your lifestyle to slow or reverse the effects of aging on your physical abilities, health, and mental agility.

RESEARCH RESULTS

> **Longitudinal studies**—*observe the same group of subjects over a long period of time, such as decades*
> **Cross-sectional studies**—*observe subjects of all ranges of ages, lifestyles, etc. at one particular time*

Many longitudinal studies indicate that aging is *not* synonymous with the decline of mental abilities. Some tests indicate that older adults in their 70s take more time and are not as accurate as participants in their 20s or 30s. However, you must remember that these are generalities and hide the fact that the physical and mental abilities of individuals differ tremendously from person to person. Informally, you know this yourself—you have friends who are physically active, other friends who are very agile mentally, and some friends who are both.

You can learn a great deal from both types of studies. Generalizations from the results of these studies often have been published indicating that the older we get, the slower and more forgetful we get. Nevertheless, within the studies are individual differences:

- All people do not age physically and mentally at the same rate.
- Not all people get more forgetful with age.
- For individuals who are over the age of 50, some mental abilities remain constant, some decrease, and some increase.

- Older persons who keep active and stimulated may improve their scores on intelligence tests.
- Some studies indicate that there may be no decline in cognitive abilities.

The Berlin Aging Study, a study of 75- to 105-year-olds living in West Berlin, shows that some of those who were 85 to 105 years old showed higher levels of performance than individuals in the 70-to-84-year-old age group. In another study, Douglas Powell tested the math and reading-comprehension skills of more than 1,500 persons. The subjects ranged in age from 25 to 92 years old. He found that 25 percent to 33 percent of subjects in their 80s performed as well as the younger participants. Moreover, even the lowest scorers exhibited only small declines that did not interfere with daily living. Powell coined the term *optimal agers* to describe a small fraction of those in their 80s and 90s who exhibited exceptional scores, placing them near the top of mental abilities for all ages.

The MacArthur Studies of Successful Aging identified four traits common to those people who are most likely to remain mentally sharp and active. They

- Are better educated
- Are more physically active
- Have better lung capacity
- Possess higher self-efficacy

Many other longitudinal and cross-sectional studies have attempted to determine those characteristics that make some individuals optimal agers. Dr. K. Warner Schaie began the Seattle Longitudinal Study in 1956. Since that time, he has followed more than 5,000 people. Every seven years, he interviews and tests them to determine their progress and declines, if any. He has determined that various characteristics are associated with an individual's ability to maintain mental agility and alertness:

- An absence of cardiovascular and other diseases
- A high socioeconomic status

- Involvement in a complex and intellectually stimulating environment
- A flexible personality at midlife
- The high cognitive status of a spouse
- Maintenance of high levels of perceptual processing speed

This is a huge chapter. This, along with Chapter 7, "Enjoy Your Ageless Mental Agility," is one of the two big How-to-Fix-It chapters. You will learn how to use the information you acquired in the previous chapters to get your body ready to support an Agile Mind.

You will learn how to implement the changes necessary to build a brawny brain and understand precisely how these changes will support an agile brain. So while you are reading, notice which techniques you already use (and congratulate yourself), pick a few new ideas to incorporate, and above all else, keep learning! (You'll know why we said that later.)

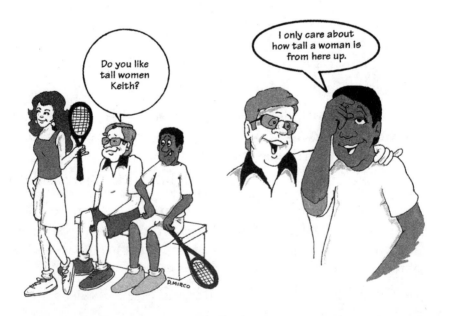

RHYTHMS OF YOUR BRAIN

Our mind, spirit, and body perform an intricate, intensely interactive dance of life. When our body's health is compromised, as when we have a cold, our cognitive functions and emotional well-being suffer. When we suffer an emotional upset, our judgments are not as clear as we would like, and sometimes our body rebels under the stress with gastrointestinal flareups or other aches and pains. In addition, when our cognitive functioning is not up to par, we cannot control or respond correctly to the physical and emotional demands in our environment.

One of the central controlling mechanisms in this dance of life is the natural rhythm of our bodies. It causes us to wake at approximately the same hour each morning, coordinates blood pressure and temperature cycles, and controls hundreds of activities within our bodies. These rhythms can be a tremendous influence on our emotional well-being, physical functioning, and cognitive abilities. How effective we are at improving our bodies and minds while fighting off diseases and age-related changes depends to various degrees on our health, age, genetics, gender, attitude, and natural rhythms. The body's natural rhythms are classified as

- **Ultradian,** which are shorter than 24-hour cycles, such as the rhythm of your heartbeat
- **Circadian,** which are approximately 24-hour cycles, such as your sleep/wake pattern
- **Infradian,** which are longer than circadian, as in a woman's hormonal cycle
- **Seasonal,** which cycle throughout the year, as in a man's testosterone cycle

The emphasis in this book is on circadian rhythms unless otherwise noted. These rhythms are of a good length, so we can easily see the effects of interventions. In addition, many of these rhythms directly and indirectly affect our mental capability.

Circadian Rhythm Revisited

Circadian is from the Latin word *circa*, meaning *about*, and *dies*, meaning *day*. The structure in our bodies that serves as our biological clock is called the *supra chiasmatic nucleus* (SCN). See Figure 6-1.

> *Our biological clock is the* supra chiasmatic nucleus *(SCN).*

Located in the hypothalamus, a quarter–sized structure in the brain, the SCN is vital for the formation of long-term

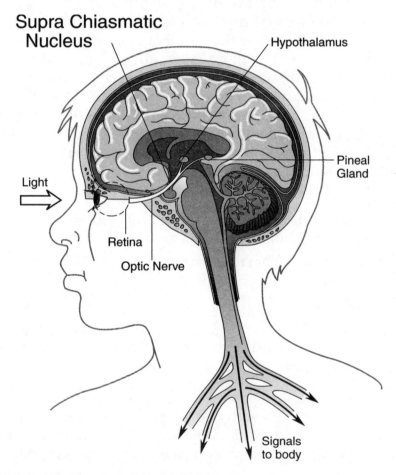

Figure 6-1 Supra chiasmatic nucleus

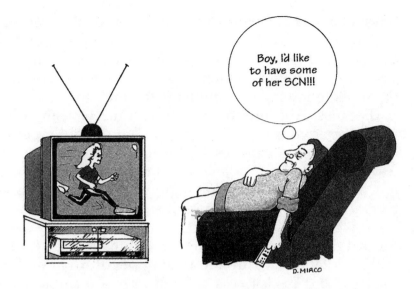

memories. Light reaches the retina of the eye, travels via the optic nerve to the brain, and resets the SCN.

The resulting change in the SCN produces cycles, affects the nervous system, and sends signals to the pineal gland, which in turn affects hormonal levels. Recent studies indicate that the SCN can be reset using exposure to light on other areas of the body, such as the back of the knees, where blood vessels are close to the surface of the skin.

Your body temperature, blood pressure, hormonal levels, sleep/wake cycle, and many other functions are controlled by your particular circadian rhythm. Although your rhythms may be similar to someone else's in many respects, they will not be an exact match. Scientists have performed experiments that demonstrate how much control the SCN has over a body. In animals, if the SCN of one animal is replaced with the SCN from a second animal, the first animal will take on the biological rhythms of the second animal.

We intentionally or unintentionally interfere with the functioning of our internal clocks in many ways. When *Daylight Savings Time* (DST) goes into effect in the spring, the clocks in your house may be easily reset, but the clocks in your body are a little more difficult to reset. For several days, you may have difficulty going to sleep and getting up at the proper time, because it is one full hour earlier than it had been. You may find yourself more irritable in the mornings. In fact, traffic accidents increase by 8 percent during the week following DST implementation.[1]

Because exposure to sunlight is a mechanism you can use to reset your circadian rhythm, you might go outside each morning to help reset your internal clock. Nevertheless, until your body adjusts, be careful and don't schedule any important activities that require your peak mental concentration early in the morning.

Traveling across multiple time zones (especially moving toward the east) also disrupts our internal clocks. It can result in irritability, gastrointestinal upset, drowsiness during the day, and restlessness at night. These symptoms of a disharmonious biological rhythm often are referred to as *jet lag*. Some hotels now offer special rooms with full-spectrum lights that you can use to reset your internal clock.

> **Full-spectrum lighting**—*Standard incandescent bulbs do not produce the blue end of the color spectrum, and florescent bulbs often miss out on the red end. Full-spectrum light bulbs produce all the colors of the rainbow and generate light similar to natural sunlight.*

Glenn Austin uses a mental trick to minimize jet lag. Whenever he flies into another time zone, as soon as he gets on the plane, he adjusts his watch to the destination time. If he falls asleep on the plane, all the better—he wakes up in the new time.

Rotating shift work also results in the same jet-lag type of symptoms as our bodies try to adjust to continually changing systems of work and rest. Your body has numerous internal rhythms synchronized within a daily pattern. Jet lag and rotating shift work can desynchronize your internal clocks. Sleep, blood pressure, body temperature, and other cyclic functions can become out of phase with each other. It takes several days for the body to readjust and reestablish your natural rhythms. Moreover, remember from Chapter 2 that we need proper sleep patterns to assist us with our memory formations and cognitive functions (more on that in just a bit).

Your emotions can affect your body's cycles. Blood pressure has its own circadian rhythm, decreasing while you sleep and rising when you awaken. Those people with higher levels of anger and hostility lose this natural lowering of blood pressure during the night hours. This elevated blood pressure increases the risk of heart attack, organ damage, and stroke. Don't go to bed upset. You can do a nice little exercise whenever you have difficulty sleeping because you are stressed or otherwise upset:

1. Lie calmly on the bed.
2. Begin at the top of your head. Concentrate to see whether you can contract your scalp. Tighten, hold for a second or two, and then release.
3. Move to the back of your head. Tighten, hold, and then release your scalp.
4. Move to your forehead. Tighten the skin, hold, and then release.
5. Move to your eyebrows. Tighten the brows, hold, and then release.
6. Move to your nose. Tighten the nose, hold, and then release.
7. Move to your ears. Tighten the ears, hold, and then release.
8. Move to your lips. Tighten the lips, hold, and then release.
9. Continue the process down to your toes, taking small steps along the way. Include each finger as a step, each muscle in your arms, one arm at a time, one muscle at a time.

(Author's note: I have never been able to do this with my toes. I have always fallen asleep before then. It's a *very* relaxing exercise my father taught me!)

It is common knowledge that the risk of heart attack is highest in the morning when you wake up. But this is the time when the level of many medicines taken to reduce the risk of heart attack is at its lowest. Other diseases, such as arthritis and even the common cold, have general times of the day when sufferers expect symptoms to be at their maximum levels. Medicines to counteract these diseases should be matched to biological rhythms. Proper timing of medications increases effectiveness, decreases side effects, allows you to manage your condition better, and may allow you to take smaller doses. Later, we have a section devoted to your medications and the effects they can have on your cognitive abilities. Perhaps if you can reduce the dosage using more efficient administration techniques, you can minimize the effects on your mental processes. Do not attempt to reduce the dosage of prescription medicines, however, without consulting with your physician first.

As an example, compare the general pain cycles of osteoarthritis, the most common form of arthritis, and rheumatoid arthritis. Those suffering from osteoarthritis and those suffering from rheumatoid arthritis often take the same nonsteroidal anti-inflammatory remedy, such as Ibuprofen, to alleviate their pain. Those with osteoarthritis tend to have more pain in the evening than in the morning and should take the pain reliever around noon or midafternoon. Those suffering from rheumatoid arthritis, in which pain is higher in the morning, should take the pain reliever in the evening. Please keep in mind that these are only suggestions. If your doctor has told you to take the pain reliever at your convenience, then you might want to consider altering the time of day when you take it. However, if your doctor has told you a specific time to take your medicine, you must ask your doctor *before* you change your schedule.

Researchers already are investigating this concept of matching the timing of medication administration to the symptom cycle and call it *chronotherapy*. They predict that pharmaceutical companies, doctors, and patients will soon become familiar with this term. Medicines will need to be redesigned and prescribed differently. The body does not need a constant level of medicine in the blood throughout the day. It needs larger doses at specific times to support the body's fight against symptom changes during the day. Already, many cancer centers are timing treatments to match the circadian rhythm of the patient with excellent success rates.

Although not every researcher agrees, some research results indicate that surgeries also can be more successful if scheduled according to a person's biological rhythms. Death after surgery is three times as likely at midnight as at noon. A 20-year study of 1,200 premenopausal women found that 76 percent of those women who had surgery for breast cancer in the week after ovulation, and only 63 percent of those

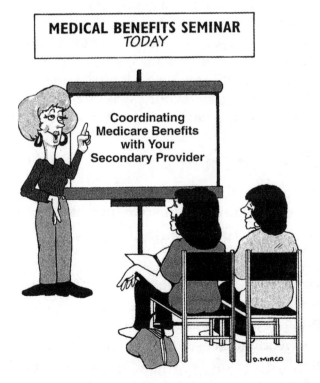

"OK, Claire. If you were saving your brain for something big, this is it."

women who had the surgery earlier in the menstrual cycle, were cancer free after five years.[2]

Just to reemphasize, be sure to ask your doctor about the best times to take your medication. Do not attempt to change the timing or dose of your medicines without the prior approval of your physician. In addition, when a doctor asks you whether your condition is worse in the morning, the doctor is probably asking you about when you wake up. If you are doing shift work and waking up in the evening, alert the doctor to this situation before answering that question. And for all you people out there who have experienced major difficulties with medical insurance claims, think of it as an excellent learning experience exercising those interpersonal, intrapersonal, linguistic, mathematical, and logical intelligences.

This information about your body's natural rhythms is important to both your physical and mental abilities. You need to be aware of the effects of your natural rhythms on your body in order to minimize stress, perhaps decrease the amount of medicine you take, increase your resistance to disease, and help regulate your sleep. All these factors are discussed in greater detail throughout the rest of this chapter.

RESTING YOUR BRAIN

Before you read the information regarding sleep, answer the following questions about your current sleep patterns:

1. How many hours a night, on average, do you sleep? _____

2. How many hours a night, on average, do you lie awake in bed? _____

3. When you wake in the mornings, do you feel refreshed and ready to get started on a new day? _____

4. If you take a nap or naps during the day, how many hours, on average, do you sleep? _____

5. On a scale of 1 to 5, with 1 being excellent and 5 being extremely poor, how would you rate your sleep habits?

_____

Sleep deprivation results in fatigue (no surprise there), irritability, decreased attention span, slower response time, memory gaps, and impaired judgment. Sleep is essential to maintain memory functions. There are two primary types of sleep: _rapid eye movement_ (REM) sleep, during which you dream, and non-REM, or slow-wave sleep. The sleep cycle can be divided into stages that you cycle through approximately every 90 minutes (an ultradian rhythm). Non-REM sleep accounts for 75 percent of your sleep and has four stages. As you progress through the stages, sleep becomes deeper and brain waves become larger. After you reach the deepest level of sleep in stage four, sleep begins to lighten until you reach REM sleep. It appears that different types of learning may be facilitated within the different types of sleep, (See Figure 6-2).

During REM sleep, activity in the brain begins in the pons and other midbrain areas. The pons communicates with the cerebral cortex and the thalamus. The pons also "turns off" motor neurons in the spinal cord, preventing movement.

REM sleep is important to procedural memory formation of tasks such as typing and playing the piano. People who learned a repetitive task were found to be more efficient at the task after sleeping and experiencing REM sleep. In one study, subjects were trained on a task in the evening. During the night, some of the subjects were awakened each time they entered REM sleep, and the rest were awakened each time they entered non-REM sleep. Those who were awakened during REM sleep were just as efficient as they were the evening before. However, those who were awakened during non-REM sleep demonstrated significant improvement in performance over the performance levels of the evening before.[3] Another type of memory, called _declarative_, in which

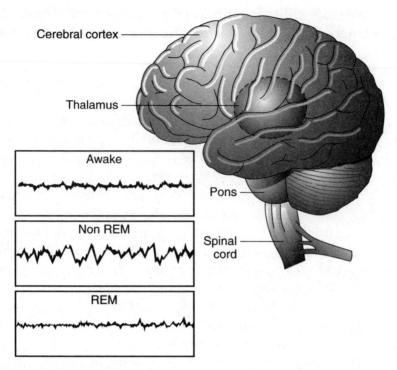

Figure 6-2 Different types of sleep

memories are formed for events such as the vacation you took, people you visited, and conversations you had, also requires REM sleep for consolidation of information.

Recall from earlier chapters that REM sleep makes it possible to transfer new learning to long-term memory. REM sleep occurs earlier and lasts longer for individuals who have participated in intense learning experiences. REM sleep is a required part of the learning process during which the brain's memories are replayed and compacted to conserve space. This allows the brain to conserve space more efficiently. As a point of interest, animals that do not possess the capability for REM sleep, like dolphins, have disproportionately larger brains.

The hippocampus also becomes involved as potential memories encountered during the day and determined to be important enough to store are transferred to long-term memory. One research study used mice to explore the learning process. When mice were introduced to a new environment, the hippocampus' nerve cells began firing. That night, while the mice were in non-REM sleep, the neurons in the hippocampus began to fire again in the same pattern experienced earlier in the day, but in shorter, faster bursts. And like an echo from a canyon wall, the cortex responded with neurons firing in a responsive similar pattern.[4]

In Chapter 4, you learned that patients under the influence of anesthesia and exposed to word associations on a recording could recall a statistically significant number of the associations. Another study involved participants who learned a complex logic task while an auditory signal, a clicking noise, occurred in the background. During REM sleep after the learning experience, some members of the group were re-exposed to the clicking noise and some were not. Those exposed to the same auditory stimuli during REM sleep retained the information 23 percent better than the group that did not hear the clicking noise during REM sleep. Do you remember the theory of playing records while you sleep to learn a foreign language or other material? The processing of information continues while we are asleep. So, not only do we process events we have experienced throughout the day, but we can subconsciously add to these memories. Many health professionals recommend that loved ones talk to unconscious patients with words of encouragement and support to aid the healing process. And how many of us have soothed a fretful baby back to sleep before he fully wakens by whispering words of love and comfort?

As we age, many people experience a disruption of natural rhythms, especially sleep patterns. We also experience changes in our alertness rhythm, especially men. This could be related to the fact that men experience shorter REM cycles, wake up more frequently, and experience less slow-wave sleep. Women do not seem to suffer as much disruption as men. Another change in natural rhythms accounts for a shift in sleeping times. Elders tend to be more alert in the morning and become drowsier in the afternoon.[5]

Insomnia is trouble falling or staying asleep and is considered chronic when the symptoms last for more than three weeks. After even one night of interrupted sleep, people complain of irritability, shorter attention span, memory gaps, and impaired judgment. Insomnia can exacerbate these symptoms. More than 50 percent of chronic insomnia cases can be attributed to emotional stress such as depression or anxiety. Typically, depression causes you to awaken early, whereas anxiety may prevent you from going to sleep. Pain, restlessness, or other symptoms of illnesses also can disrupt your sleeping patterns.

Moreover, once your sleep is disrupted, learned insomnia can keep you awake until the pattern is broken. My mother experienced learned insomnia after she moved to the country. The barking of her dog at foraging nocturnal animals would awaken her. She then would get out of bed to check on the dog, and since she was awake, she would treat herself to something sweet to eat. Before too long, she was waking up at about that hour of the night regardless of whether the dog was barking. Her body had "learned" to wake up at an inappropriate time. Irregular sleep patterns, such as staying up late and sleeping in on the weekends, also can disrupt your sleep patterns. In addition, some medications can work on the central nervous system and prevent restful sleep from occurring.

Interestingly, more than 50 percent of those people 65 years old and older experience regular disruptions of sleep cycles. Many elders do not produce sufficient quantities of melatonin or do not have sufficient melatonin receptors in the brain.[6] This inhibits the ability to initiate and maintain sleep during the night. Melatonin is produced by the pineal gland in the brain in rhythmical cycles, with high production levels at night and minute quantities produced during the day. See Figure 6-3.

Many seniors whose brains have ceased manufacturing adequate levels of melatonin can benefit from doses of melatonin approximately two hours before bedtime. Alzheimer's patients, who also have reduced levels of melatonin, bene-

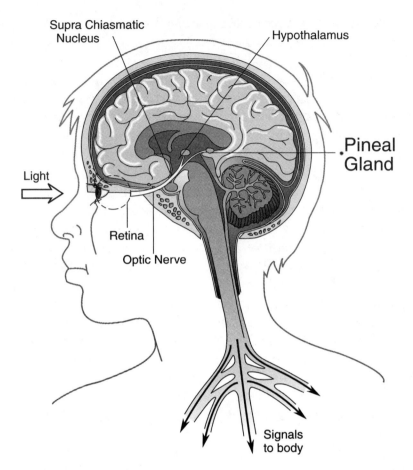

Figure 6-3 Pineal gland

fit from melatonin supplements as well. If the trouble is going to sleep, but once you fall asleep you can stay asleep, some physicians recommend fast-release melatonin supplements. If you have trouble staying asleep, a controlled-release form of melatonin may help. It may take several days to a week before you see an improvement and begin to reinstate your natural cycle.[7] These supplements are somewhat controversial, and you should not take them without your physician's approval because of possible drug interactions and questionable quality control of many over-the-counter supplements.

Research indicates that Alzheimer's patients get less REM sleep than normal adults.

A survey of 1,400 retirees at the National Institute of Health and Medical Research in Paris discovered that half the individuals had breathing problems during sleep, such as snoring or sleep apnea. Approximately 44 percent of older adults also experience *periodic limb movement in sleep* (PLMS). Symptoms are leg movements and kicks repeated every 20 to 40 seconds throughout the night. Each movement causes the person to arouse enough to prevent restful sleep.[8]

When your internal clock goes off schedule, sleeping cycles suffer. Sleep is a critical ingredient in the learning process and in our ability to recall information later. "When apnea led to daytime sleepiness, researchers found, the person showed significant loss of short-term memory and alertness on psychological test, the kind of mental slippage that can lead to dementia." Sonia Ancoli-Israel, Director of the Sleep Disorders Clinic at San Diego's Veterans Administration Hospital says, "If you treated sleep problems in people with mild dementia, I think there's a chance their mental deterioration would improve."[9]

If you suffer from insomnia, you might check with your physician and pharmacist about possible side effects of your medications that may interfere with your sleep cycle. Some drugs, such as some beta-blockers prescribed for hypertension, interfere with the production of melatonin in the brain. Others may interfere with its absorption. Perhaps you can have your doctor prescribe a different type of drug that will not interfere with your production or absorption of melatonin.

Some people use alcohol as an aide to go to sleep. It does relax you initially, but several hours later, when the alcohol is depleted, it results in insomnia. You can use other techniques to induce relaxation and help you fall asleep.

Can't Sleep? Try These Tips:

Plan to avoid insomnia.

Don't watch TV or read before going to bed.

Get some physical exercise during the day.

Avoid caffeine, alcohol, and tobacco.

Avoid illuminated bedroom clocks.

Keep your bed a place for sleep.

Don't sleep late on weekends.

Get up earlier in the morning.

Keep regular bedtime hours.

Sleep on a good, firm bed.

Get a body massage.

Visualize something peaceful.

Visualize something boring.

Imagine it's time to get up.

If you can't sleep, get up.

Try progressive relaxation.

Count happy thoughts.

Rub your stomach.

Eat a bedtime snack.

Sleep on your back.

Wiggle your toes.

Take a warm bath.

Drink warm milk.

Listen to music.

Breathe deeply.

—list compiled by Oufei Zhao

Not only do you need to get adequate sleep each night, you need to have a regular sleep schedule from day to day. Some helpful hints used in an eldercare facility to facilitate maintenance of a proper sleep schedule may be helpful for you as well:[10]

- If physically possible, do not remain in bed for more than one hour when not sleeping. Remaining in bed may confuse your circadian sleep/wake cycle.

- Establish and follow a regular wake/sleep cycle. Try to get to bed about the same time each night except on special occasions.

- Match roommates' night and day routines as closely as possible. You may not have a roommate, per se, but if your spouse or other family members keep a different schedule than you, it may interfere with your ability to maintain an uninterrupted sleep cycle.

- No matter how tired or depressed you may be, get out of bed and get busy. You must tire yourself a little in order to be ready for sleep at bedtime.

- Avoid caffeine in beverages, chocolates, and medications. Read the labels. You will be surprised at what has caffeine in it, especially medications.

- Keep the facilities as bright as possible during the day. It will help your overall attitude and literally brighten your day. If you can open the window shades and get some sun, it will assist your circadian rhythms.

- Keep rooms as dark as possible during the night. It will assist you in staying asleep once you get to that blessed state.

- Minimize nighttime noise and disturbances.

- Limit naps to one per day for a maximum of 30 minutes each. If you sleep too much during the day, you will not be ready to sleep at night. Remember how you have to keep little babies up during the day so they will sleep at night if their schedule gets off.

- Encourage clients to go outside and get as much exposure to sunlight as possible. You may need help resetting that biological clock in order to rest.

Because sleep is so essential to your mental capability and quality of life, we tried to include brief descriptions of as many disruptions to a good, restful sleep as possible. You may have found some information about sleep that pertains directly to you. If you rated your sleep satisfaction as a 3, 4, or 5, did you discover any suggestions that might help you to achieve a higher quality of sleep?

FEEDING YOUR BRAIN

You know that proper nutrition assists your body to fight infection, prevent cancer, and function efficiently during daily activities. Take just a few minutes to evaluate your diet. In the blank next to each food category, write the number of servings you eat on a typical day:

_____ Fruit
_____ Vegetables
_____ Meat/Poultry
_____ Milk, Yogurt, Cheese
_____ Bread, Cereal, Rice, Pasta
_____ Meats, Poultry, Fish, Dry Beans, Eggs, Nuts
_____ Fats, Oils, Sweets

The brain requires 25 percent of the body's available resources.

You must keep your body adequately nourished to provide the essential nutrients in sufficient quantities. After all, the brain takes 25 percent of the available resources, and if what is available is not enough, 25 percent of "not enough" is still "not enough." You may need to learn compensation strategies to maintain your body fitness and function at peak performing capacity. Reducing the energy drain on total available resources increases the amount of resources available for mental processes. Let's start with proper nutrition. Like a car, you need a good supply and quality of fuel to run efficiently and at peak capacity.

Plan a Day's Meals Based on the USDA Food Pyramid

If you have lived in the United States in the past decade, you probably are very familiar with the Food Guide Pyramid released by the U.S. Department of Agriculture (refer to Figure 4-5). It is on many food containers you purchase in the grocery stores. The admonitions are clear: Eat a certain number of foods from each of the tiers of the pyramid each day.

This is because the body needs more than 40 nutrients, and no one food supplies them all. If you just glance at the pyramid, it appears impossible to accommodate all of the recommendations in a single day. It may take some practice, but it is doable!

Use these guidelines to select food for a typical day. Several of the tiers recommend a range of servings. If you are slight in build, choose the lower of the number ranges. If you are big boned, select the higher. For example, we should eat two to four servings of fruit per day. Small people should choose two, and large people should choose four.

Complete the chart below: (We have filled in the morning snack as an example for you.)

Meals	Bread, Cereal, Rice Pasta (6–11)	Vegetables (3–5)	Fruit (2–4)	Milk, Yogurt, Cheese (2–3)	Meats, Poultry, Fish, Dry Beans, Eggs, Nuts (2–3)	Fats, Oils, Sweets (sparingly)
Breakfast						
Snack		1 carrot		1 glass of milk		
Lunch						
Snack						
Dinner						
Snack						

The brain uses biochemicals to perform cognitive functions. It extracts these biochemicals from the foods we eat. Various biochemicals are used to make you feel happy, angry, relaxed, stressed, energized, or calm. Certain neurotransmitters, such as serotonin, assist with sleep regulation and anxiety reduction. Serotonin is manufactured from the amino acid tryptophan, which is found in protein-rich foods. Let's take a little time to discuss just a few of the neurotransmitters.

Acetylcholine is one of the essential ingredients for memory formation and maintenance. Acetylcholine is made from the fat-like B vitamin choline, which is found in egg yolks and organ meats. Scientists do not fully understand the manufacturing process but do know that Alzheimer's disease can be linked to the underproduction of acetylcholine due to the destruction of the cholinergic neurons that make it. Very few studies have been done on the effects of choline, but the few that do exist indicate that choline supplementation does enhance memory and reduce fatigue. However, if you have an abundant supply of choline and do not use it, this is similar to having a full tank of gasoline and not driving your car. You must use your mind to make the choline work for you.

Soldiers have been given tyrosine supplements and then exposed to environmental stresses such as high altitudes or prolonged cold. The typical responses to these conditions, headaches and memory lapses, are reduced. This study also indicates the importance of these biochemicals to the proper working mechanisms of the brain.

Other neurotransmitters, collectively called *catecholamines*, control arousal and anxiety states and are major factors in the brain's ability to handle stress. You may have heard of some of these: dopamine, epinephrine, and norepenephrine. Dopamine and norepenephrine are derived from the amino acid tyrosine. Stress in your environment depletes your blood of tyrosine, which is an important player in the manufacture of neurotransmitters. Amino acids, which are found in protein-rich foods and other dietary substances, are used by the body to create these neurotransmitters.

Deficiencies of B vitamins result in profound deleterious effects on the brain, such as abnormal brain waves, impaired memory, higher levels of anxiety and confusion, irritability, and depression. Even marginal deficiency levels demonstrate these effects. Remember serotonin? Folic acid is required to maintain the proper levels of serotonin in your brain. If your

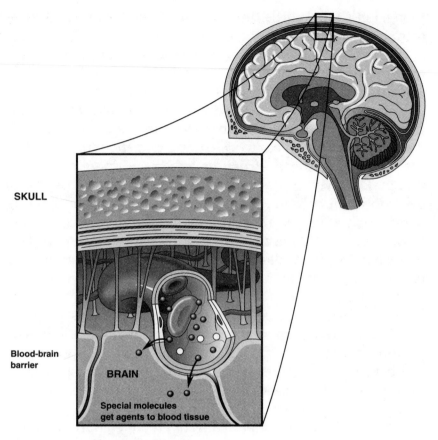

SKULL

Blood-brain
barrier

BRAIN

Special molecules
get agents to blood tissue

Figure 6-4 Blood–brain barrier

thiamin (B1) supply is deficient, your brain's ability to use glucose is reduced, and less energy is available for your brain to maintain mental activities.

From these few examples, it is obvious that if deficits exist because of aging or stress, supplementation improves cognitive functioning. However, there is no evidence that any positive results will come from supplements if normal amounts of the neurotransmitters already exist. And there is always the possibility that if you self-prescribe supplements, you could overdose, resulting in adverse, possibly dangerous, reactions. A natural competition exists for elements crossing the blood-brain barrier in the blood supply.

Supplementing certain amino acids could overload your system and keep other necessary precursor amino acids from crossing into your brain. So do not run out and buy amino acid supplements.

The best way to supplement your body's natural require-ments is by following a balanced diet.

The Dieting Trap

Many people fall into the trap of dieting. Cutting back on the *quantity* of food and not changing the *quality* of the food actually is detrimental to your weight-maintenance pro-gram. The following lighthearted quiz is a matching exercise for some of the not-too-successful diets. Match each ill-fated diet with its name.

a. Seafood diet	_____ Never say diet.
b. Light diet	_____ I never 'et a food I didn't like.
c. Sir Edmund Hillary diet	_____ Ohhhhnnhhhh . . . I'm hungggrrryyy.
d. Will Rogers diet	_____ I watch my food all the way from my plate to my lips.
e. I Watch What I Eat diet	_____ As soon as it gets light, I start eating.
f. Wine diet	_____ I see food, I eat it.
g. Fondue diet	_____ I ate it because it was there.
h. James Bond diet	_____ Cheeze, I'm hungry.

The matching game above is an exercise for your linguis-tic intelligence. All of the answers are a result of word play.

a. The Seafood diet   I see food, I eat it.
   Words that sound alike.

b. The Light diet   As soon as it gets light, I start eating.
   Two meanings for the same word.

c. Sir Edmund Hillary diet   I ate it because it was there.
   When asked why he had climbed Mt. Everest, Sir Hillary said "Because it was there."

d. Will Rogers diet   I never 'et a food I didn't like.
   A famous quote of Rogers is "I never met a man I didn't like".

e. I watch what I eat diet   I watch my food all the way from my plate to my lips.
   Two meanings for the same word.

f. The Wine Diet   Ohhhhhmmmhhh—I'm hungggrrryyy.
   Wine and whine sound alike.

g. The Fondue diet   Cheeze, I'm hungry.
   Fondue is a cheese dish. Cheese and cheeze sound alike.

h. The James Bond Diet   Never say diet.
   One of the James Bond stories is named "Never Say Die." Words that sound alike.

It is important for you to eat a balanced diet. Not only does it keep your body healthy, but it keeps your mind supplied with the nutrients necessary to function at peak capacity. For a general rule of thumb, anything brightly colored is brain food (just as crunchy fruits and vegetables, in general, are anticancer foods). You will learn in the next chapter how to fine-tune your mental processes and regain the mental agility you possessed 15 to 20 years ago. If you do not get adequate sleep and properly fuel your body to support these new practices, however, you will not reap your fullest benefits.

Anything brightly colored is brain food.

Calculate Your Body Mass Index

Perhaps you are worried that you are eating too much or too little. All of us worry at one time or another about our proportions. Garfield, the popular cartoon cat created by Jim Davis, has a unique perspective on the weight issue and quips, "I'm not overweight. I'm undertall." But seriously, there is a calculation you can do to compare your height and weight.

Let's use a little old-fashioned math (exercise those particular brain cells!) and determine one of the factors of your physical health: a measurement called your *Body Mass Index* (BMI). Healthy older adults have a body mass index of 22 to 27. The calculation warrants use of a calculator. Here's the formula:

$$BMI = \frac{704 \times (\text{your weight})}{(\text{your height})^2}$$

Here are the steps:

1. Using a calculator, key in 704.
2. Press the multiplication sign.
3. Key in your weight in pounds.
4. Press the division key.
5. Key in your height in inches. (If you are 5'2"tall, that's 62 inches.)
6. Press the division key.
7. Key in your height in inches again.
8. Press the equal key.

The number in the display is your Body Mass Index. If the number is less than 22 or more than 27, you may want to talk to your doctor about your results.

EXERCISING YOUR BRAIN

Everyone is well aware of some of the benefits of regular exercise. It tones the body and helps you maintain a proper weight. It also helps to prevent osteoporosis, takes years off your physical age, and can improve your memory and intelligence performance.

A study was performed with rats in which some were not allowed to exercise, some ran on a wheel (comparable to people on a treadmill), and some were taught to navigate an obstacle course. The rats that ran on the wheel grew more blood vessels to supply the brain, and the rats that ran the obstacle course showed increased growth in brain cells. The best type of physical exercise is one that exercises both the mind and the body.[11] Tennis requires physical exertion combined with mental strategy and so is an excellent example.

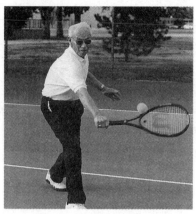

Photo courtesy of Henry Ortega

Older and Wiser

Leo LeBorde is a 79-year-old veteran of the tennis court. He plays the Senior Tennis Circuit and coaches the younger students. His wife, who is 14 years his junior, describes him as not only extremely healthy and very rarely ill but as extremely quick witted. She can never "best" him at verbal repartee. I have told him that I want him to coach me, as I have decided to take up tennis after meeting him!

Another superb example is square dancing. Square dancing requires concentration and mental attention to the dance while physically interacting with others. Later in this chapter, we discuss why social interactions also are critical to the retention of your mental abilities. Walking with a friend also can provide you with exercise, social interaction, and mental stimulation.

Let's discuss two types of exercise: aerobic and resistance training. Examples of aerobic exercise are *calisthenics* (from the Greek word for *beautiful strength*), rapid walking, running, dancing, hiking, and so on. *Aerobic* refers to the expanded use of oxygen by your body as you perform these exercises. Participating in this type of activity increases heart and lung fitness, overall endurance, and flexibility—but not strength. It also increases the amount of oxygen delivered to the brain.

The National Institute of Aging conducted a study using 65- to 75-year-olds. After beginning aerobic workouts and maintaining them for approximately three months, a 25 percent improvement in decision-making tasks and responding to visual and auditory cues was demonstrated.

In addition, engaging in regular, high levels of physical activity counteracts the natural breakdown of the circadian rhythm as we age.[12] Low or medium levels of activity are not sufficient to counteract the effect of aging on the rest-activity rhythm. To counteract the effects of age on your rest-activity rhythm, you need a higher level of activity.

Perhaps you want to start a little slower than aerobics. Don't think that just because you don't feel comfortable with aerobics—yet—you can't do anything at all. Numerous studies of men and women of all ages show that those who exercise live longer than those who are sedentary. One long walk each week can take one year off your biological age. A study of 40,000 women in Iowa revealed that just taking one long walk a week can reduce the rate of death by 12 percent, compared to all sedentary women. Jogging, swimming, and other more vigorous activities increase health and reduce the risk even more.[13]

Resistance exercise, such as weight training, increases the size and strength of your muscles but does not improve endurance. Resistance training of 66-year-old men, training at 80 percent of maximum level for 12 weeks, increased strength approximately 5 percent each day. You don't even have to be in good physical shape to start.

A progressive resistance training program that lasted eight weeks and met three times each week was designed for institutionalized, invalid elders in their 90s. Weight lifting improved their muscle strength 175 percent, while the cross-sectional area of muscle increased 15 percent, and their walking speed increased by 50 percent. Some even began to walk

without using a cane! The increased muscle strength facilitated moving from sitting to standing and climbing stairs.
Also, incidences of falling when moving from a chair were
reduced. After the initial training period, the elders retained
the results of the training with only one lifting session a
week. If weight lifting can so drastically improve the condition of institutionalized adults in their nineties, imagine what
it can do for you!

Amazingly, in the age group of older seniors, only 5 percent of men and 1 percent of women participate in weight
training.[14] Perhaps few people try weight lifting because
they are not aware of the benefits and the ease of getting
started. You do not have to go to a gym.

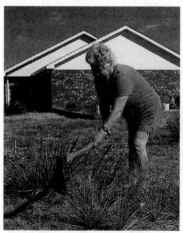

Photo courtesy of Henry Ortega

Older and Wiser

*Virginia Chestnut has had an adventurous three years. Three
years ago at 78 years of age, she sold the family home, moved into
a house in the country that she designed herself, and has since had
several operations to clear blocked arteries. And despite the
changes (or perhaps because of all the new experiences), you will
never meet a more determined, full-of-life senior!*

Dr. Wetzel's dad, Buford Chestnut, used heavy weights he made himself to perform leg lifts while seated in a chair. You could start by using canned goods or plastic milk bottles filled with water as lifting weights for the arms, or go outside and hoe the garden. Virginia Chestnut participates in resistance exercises, although she wouldn't describe it as such. She uses a hoe that weighs 7.5 pounds. You can see her just about any warm day chopping down yucca plants in the Texas panhandle.

Another excellent benefit of exercising is an increase in arterial flexibility. The arteries of adults who exercise regularly can expand more than the arteries of sedentary individuals. This is an important quality and may reduce the severity and damaging effects in case of a heart attack. It also helps to transport more nutrients and oxygen to the brain.

Always be sure to warm up and cool down when exercising. One excellent method is walking in place for three to five minutes. Even those who are in good shape can experience cardiac abnormalities without a proper warmup or cooldown. If any of the following symptoms of physical distress occur while you are exercising, *stop immediately* and seek medical attention:[15]

- Excessive overheating
- Feeling lightheaded or dizzy
- Rapid breathing that doesn't slow down
- Any type of chest pain
- Pain, bruising, or bleeding

The Surgeon General's Report

Adults reap many benefits from exercise, because it

- Enhances the ability to do daily tasks
- Improves outlook and attitude
- Relieves stress

- Burns calories
- Maintains

    Muscular strength
    Joint structure
    Joint function

- Improves

    Balance
    Posture
    The condition of the heart
    The condition of the lungs
    The condition of the blood vessels

- Reduces

    Risk of falling
    Rate of bone loss in women with osteoporosis
    Risk of having a heart attack
    Blood pressure in people with hypertension
    Risk of developing non–insulin dependent diabetes
    Risk of developing colon cancer
    Depression
    Anxiety

- Prevents or delays high blood pressure
- Prevents or relieves constipation
- May improve body-fat distribution
- May help rebuild bone density
- May reduce the rate of bone calcium loss in post-menopausal women who don't take estrogen

The Surgeon General's Report — Conclusions

- Inactive people can improve their health and well-being by becoming moderately active on a regular basis.
- Physical activity need not be strenuous to achieve health benefits.

- Greater health benefits can be achieved by increasing the amount (duration, frequency, or intensity) of physical activity.

Moderate Physical Activity

Uses 150 calories per day or 1,000 calories per week

Activity	Minutes to Perform Activity to Burn 150 Calories
Washing and waxing car	45–60
Washing windows or floors	45–60
Walking 1-3/4 miles	35
Walking 2 miles	30
Running 1-1/2 miles	15
Bicycling 5 miles	30
Water aerobics	30

10 Tips For Developing an Exercise Program

Colleen Pierre, MS, RD, LN, an instructor in the Odyssey of Aging program at Johns Hopkins University, suggests this list as a safe way to begin to exercise.

1. Begin gently.

   Start at the level that's right for you. At any age, your body will respond if you coax it. If you're over 40, overweight, smoke, or have a medical condition, check with your doctor first.

2. Beginners start with every other day.

   Your body needs recovery days to rest and get stronger.

3. Increase time gradually.

   Each week, add a few minutes per day to your workout. You'll slowly get more fit, but your body will hardly notice. No pain, plenty of progress!

4. Work a little harder.

When your workout gets to be 30 minutes long, exercise a little harder for a few minutes during each workout. You'll get more fit in the same amount of time!

5. Work out a little more often.

After you're comfortable exercising three times a week for 30 to 60 minutes each time, you could increase the number of days. Choose the same or a different activity on alternate days. Follow "beginner's" rules: Start gently, increase slowly.

6. Cross train.

Develop more than one activity so you don't overuse one set of muscles and cause pain or an injury, and so you don't get bored. Learn a different activity, or learn a sport for each season of the year. Ice skate in winter. Roller blade in summer.

7. Have a foul weather plan.

Bad weather's no excuse. Join a health club, walk at a shopping mall, buy a jump rope, get an exercise video from the library, or buy a piece of indoor equipment.

8. Buy good shoes.

If you walk, run, do aerobics, or play racquet sports, good shoes keep you comfortable and prevent injuries.

9. Be sure your equipment fits.

If you ride a bicycle, ski, or use indoor equipment, have a professional check the fit. You'll be more comfortable and enjoy your activity more.

10. Listen to your body.

Take a day off when your body is really too tired to exercise, or if you're having constant pains. But get back on track after a couple of days of rest. If the pain doesn't go away, see your doctor.

Regular physical activity can cure a multitude of ills. It reduces depression and sleeplessness, lowers blood pressure, reduces the risk of heart attack and many cancers, builds healthy bones and muscles, controls weight, increases survival after surgery, and improves cognitive functions. Regular physical activity can even reduce a person's biological age by 10 to 20 years.[16] On the other hand, inactivity produces premature aging, increased risk of chronic and disabling diseases, earlier loss of independence, and earlier mortality. Surprisingly, 29 percent of seniors 65 years and older get no exercise of any sort.[17]

FEELING WITH YOUR BRAIN

Recall that your body, spirit, and mind are all interacting in a dance of life. Your emotions are very influential in the quality of your mental and physical health and efficiency. Some emotional aspects of your personality—such as a caring or loving nature, a high level of self-esteem, and a feeling of being in control of your life (self-efficacy)—are beneficial. Other emotions—such as stress, depression, and loneliness—are detrimental to the quality of your life at any age. The following assessment may help you identify how you are dealing with the highs and lows of life.

Mental-State Assessment

Ask yourself the following questions. The key to this miniquiz is *prolonged symptoms*. When you answer "yes" to any of these, be certain that the situation is characteristic for you for a period of *more than* two weeks.

1. _____ Do you feel sad most of the time for long periods of time?

2. _____ Are you irritable, and do you stay that way for more than two weeks?

3. _____ Has your weight increased or decreased without that being your intention?

4. _____ Have you experienced a change in appetite that has lasted more than two weeks?

5. _____ Are you not enjoying things you used to like to do?

6. _____ Have you had two weeks of sleepless nights, or are you sleeping more during the day?

7. _____ Do you find increased difficulty in being able to concentrate or make decisions?

8. _____ Do thoughts of death occupy your mind?

9. _____ Have others told you that they think you are behaving differently than usual?

10. _____ Do you have more than one (women) or two (men) drinks of alcohol every day?

Count the number of "yes" answers. If you responded "yes" to more than five of these, it is probably a good idea to talk to your doctor about it.

> *There is a fountain of youth: it is your mind, your talents, the creativity you bring to your life and the lives of the people you love. When you learn to tap this source, you will truly have defeated age. — Sophia Loren*

Positive creativity has myriad benefits to your well-being. But how can you become creative if you haven't had any practice doing that? Poetry is the answer. There is a simple ancient Japanese art form called the haiku *(hī cōō)*. It is characterized by the limitation that it contains exactly 17 syllables. We are proud to introduce Happy Haiku as a positive creative outlet. Happy Haiku also have exactly 17 syllables but must express a positive sentiment. A Happy Haiku from Sharon Mulgrew entitled "Happy Spring" follows.

One cherry blossom

    on tree full of buds, "Over

        here . . . like me!" Spring Starts

Take the time here to think positive thoughts connected with what you like about the other three seasons. Write a Happy Haiku about each one.

Summer ...   **Autumn ...**   **Winter ...**

After you do this (If you haven't, go back and give it a *really* good try!), visit the Web site at www.mentalagility.com to read contributions from other readers. While you are there, submit yours as well.

All you need to do to believe in what a positive creative outlook can do for you is to look at Sophia Loren, arguably the most beautiful woman on earth. We believe that most of her beauty comes from within.

Try each day to determine within yourself to have a positive outlook on life. We all have troubles, stress, and distress that we cannot control. But it is our choice how we react. By reading the next sections, you will see why it is beneficial to your mental health and agility, as well as your physical health, to promote a positive outlook on life.

Stress

Although stress is not an inescapable result of aging, most individuals suffer from some form of stress at various times of their lives. Losing a job; the loss of loved ones to death, divorce, or a debilitating illness; a decrease in safety and support structures in neighborhoods; a lack of transportation;

and a loss of independence are all stressful situations. Even happy situations, such as the birth of a baby, buying a new home, or planning parties, can be stressful.

Qualities that help people deal with stress in a positive manner are flexibility, adaptability, and a sense of humor. Also critical to the reduction of stress is a support system of people with whom you can share your distress. The ability to find meaning in stressful situations as well as just handling the problem are part of the wisdom we acquire as we age, and that experience helps us put stressful situations into perspective.[18] All these qualities and abilities reduce the negative effects of stress on our body, mind, and spirit. Neuroscientists are "convinced that people who overreact to stress lead shorter lives and are more susceptible to accelerated brain and nervous system disease."[19]

> *"A man 90 years old was asked to what he attributed his longevity. 'I reckon,' he said, with a twinkle in his eye, 'it's because most nights I went to bed and slept when I should have sat up and worried.'" — Dorothea Kent*

Stress triggers the release of hydrocortisone, which can assist you in a "fight or flight" situation by sharpening your reflexes, raising your heart rate, and preparing you to defend your life. Short-term stresses such as traffic jams or disagreements with a spouse do not seem to have long-term effects. However, long-term stressful situations such as abuse or serving in wartime situations can create permanent effects that continue years later. Months and years of elevated hydrocortisone levels can cause the hippocampus to shrink. One estimate is a 25 percent loss in mass. As Robert Sapolsky said, "This is like reporting that an emotional trauma eliminates one of the four chambers of the heart."[20] Remember that the hippocampus is essential to your abilities to concentrate, as well as to store and recall information.

Many people who are stressed lose their appetite and lose weight or eat compulsively and gain weight; as a result,

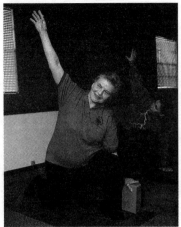

Photo courtesy of Henry Ortega

Older and Wiser

Marguerite Empie began exercising two years ago with tai chi, an excellent low-impact form of exercise. She became interested in yoga as a result. She is 79 years young and has only recently begun yoga classes. She now takes both yoga and tai chi three times a week and volunteered the information that her balance and walking have improved dramatically. She also highly values the interaction with the other class members.

they experience a decrease in *lymphocytes* (which fight off infection). An increase in psychological distress and the production of cholesterol also increases the body's production of *free radicals* (which can damage body cells and tissues).

Try massage therapy to defend yourself against the effects of stress. I know a couple in their late eighties who schedule themselves for a massage twice a month as preventative medicine. They swear they have never felt so good or had as much energy. If you do not want to go to a professional massage therapist, get together with a friend and give each other a massage. Another relaxation technique is yoga. Yoga is an ancient form of exercise that is especially beneficial for helping you learn to relax. You can start at any age.

Other negative emotions are anger, depression and loneliness. A study of 1,623 heart-attack victims, conducted by researchers at Harvard Medical School, discovered that "angry episodes" doubled the risk of a heart attack. The heart attacks "often occurred a mere two hours after the outburst."[21] Someone suffering from anger and hostility needs to learn some forms of stress management.

Loneliness is inversely related to self-esteem. Feelings of loneliness are linked to depression, anxiety, and hostility, as well as suicide and vulnerability to health problems. Patients who suffer from depression are four times more likely to die within six months of a heart attack and three times as likely to die within 10 years of a stroke. Some researchers are beginning to investigate whether treating psychological conditions can increase survival rates, and two studies show that participants in support groups have higher survival rates for various cancers. The Charles A. Dana Foundation has established the Brain-Body Connection to further research into the ramifications of this brain-body link.

Dr. Schaie found that being married to a smart spouse is directly associated with maintaining our mental abilities and aging well. He found that the mental quickness of one spouse would entice the other spouse to become more efficient in order to "keep up." Perhaps you are not married, but you may have a significant other or a close friend with whom you spend a great deal of time. You probably share some of the same interests and may have interests in different areas as well. Learn from each other. Be adventurous. Try new restaurants, take a class together, go to the movies and discuss the plot afterward over a cup of coffee. You will practice your verbal and logic skills as you converse. You will exercise "flabby" brain connections as you learn about new ideas and explore new opportunities.

To combat loneliness and mild depression, get involved. Join a senior citizens center. Take classes. Volunteer at your local elementary school, nursing home, or hospital. Helping others will help you. Your self-esteem will increase. You will have something good to look forward to. Your appetite and energy level will increase. Those brain connections will fire right and left. Reaching out to others and feeling needed is a vital part of our lives. We all want to know we have made a difference by being here on this planet. You are never too young or too old to care for others and make that difference.

Those who love deeply never grow old;
they may die of old age,
but they die young.

— Benjamin Franklin

Spiritual

A spiritual belief is linked to a higher satisfaction with life. Knowing that there is a higher plan for your life, whatever your official religion, helps you deal with stressful situations. Spirituality has been linked to successful aging. Adults who are active in religion tend to exhibit better physical and mental health than those adults who do not participate in religion as much. Religion often can provide a sense of community with other like believers who may offer the support of a family environment. Social gatherings are often a part of this sense of community and provide opportunities for you to interact and stay mentally active in a safe, caring environment.

 We believe that a sense of humor is a part of your inner spirit. Perhaps you have noticed humorous jokes and uplifting and jocular quotes throughout this book. Humor and a positive attitude are strongly associated with our feelings of being in control of our lives—whether or not we actually are. A good laugh also helps to keep us young in spirit and has been shown to be associated with aging well. Buy or check out joke books. Go out on the Internet and find joke sites. In addition, in case you're interested, you can actually search for "clean" or any other types of jokes in the library

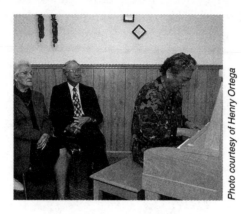

Photo courtesy of Henry Ortega

Older and Wiser

Victoria Mok is a vivacious woman full of bubbling laughter at 84 years of age. She took piano lessons as a young girl in China, but after she married and began her family of five children, Victoria did not continue to practice. As she and her husband grew old together, he often suggested that she continue playing to keep her mind sharp (he was ahead of his time). After he passed away, Victoria began playing the piano for her Sunday school class to help out and also to follow her husband's advice. She's really enjoying herself. This turns out to be a mutual benefit to her and her Sunday school class.

or on the Internet. See Appendix C, "Using the Web for Lifelong Learning," to learn how to do this. Learn to laugh and enjoy life again.

PROTECTING YOUR BRAIN

Now it is appropriate to discuss strategies for dealing with some health issues that are associated with aging—stroke, Alzheimer's disease, doctors, and medications.

As you age, it becomes more likely that you or someone you know will have a stroke, sometimes referred to as a *brain attack.* The extent of damage inflicted on an individual depends on the severity and location of the stroke, as well as the speed with which you receive treatment. The term *golden hour* was coined by Dr. R. Adams Cowley of the Maryland Institute for Emergency Medical Services, who is regarded as the pioneer of modern trauma care. Medical intervention within the first hour after trauma is critical for increasing the patient's chance of survival. This hour, called *the golden hour,* begins the moment the injury occurs. Very recent advances may have increased this window of opportunity to three hours. Nevertheless, if you think that you might be experiencing a stroke, seek help immediately. Do not delay. It is better to be safe than sorry. The effects of a stroke can be minimized with immediate attention.

Remember the discussions in Chapter 2 of where the different brain functions are located? The long-term potential for healing any damage caused by brain injury depends largely on your age. At birth, for example, both hemispheres seem to have potential for a language center. Based on observations of severely epileptic infants whose hemispheres must be surgically severed, language still can be acquired and handled in the right hemisphere. If severe damage occurs to a mature brain, the right hemisphere may not be able to accommodate speech other than an odd word here or there.

An intriguing example of the left/right hemispheres is the case of N.G., a homemaker whose corpus callosum had been severed so that no communication from one hemisphere to the other existed. Jean-Pierre Changeux describes an experiment in which objects were presented to N.G. on a split screen, so that what is presented in the left visual field is seen only by the left eye, and what is presented in the right visual field is seen by the right eye only. What the left eye sees is transmitted to the right hemisphere of the brain, and what the right eye sees is transmitted to the left hemisphere of the brain. N.G. is left-brain dominant, and therefore her language and verbal capabilities are in the left hemisphere.

When a cup was exhibited in the right visual field, the image was transmitted to N.G.'s left hemisphere and recognized. Because her verbal ability was in that side of the cortex, N.G. stated that she saw a cup. When a spoon was exhibited to her left eye, and the image was transmitted to the right hemisphere, N.G. could not verbalize the name "spoon." Instead, she could choose a spoon from a number of available objects with her left hand. The right brain identified the image to the left hand, but without the verbal abilities of the left hemisphere, N.G. could not name it. When shown a naked woman on the left side of the screen, N.G. blushed and laughed behind her hand. But when asked what she had seen, she said she had seen a flash of light. Again, she could not correctly verbalize her stimulus, but the right hemisphere recognized the image and reacted emotionally.

An acquaintance, a male engineer, had a stroke in the corpus callosum. Thus, he had trouble passing information from one hemisphere to another, as did N.G. With his emotions on one side and his math and language skills on the other, he had no trouble counting to 100 but could not answer the question "How do you feel?"

If you are dealing with the effects of a stroke, and one method does not produce improvement or recognition, keep trying other methods. If the person cannot talk, try writing. Perhaps they can sing, instead. Try presenting information from the other side or to the other hand.

Alzheimer's Disease

Interestingly (in a rather sad way), a research study reported that how we view forgetfulness depends on how old the person is that forgot the information. Both older and younger adults view forgetfulness in an older adult as a sign of senility. The same degree of forgetfulness in a younger person is considered just due to bad luck by both older and younger adult observers. A bumper sticker reads "You are never wrong until someone is listening." Isn't it a shame that we do not listen to how often we are correct and how often we remember those important facts, dates, and errands? Instead, we amplify the times we are incorrect or cannot immediately recall a desired piece of information.

Every time we forget something, it does not mean that we are entering the beginning stages of Alzheimer's. Many of us joke about Alzheimer's or senility when we cannot remember something or cannot find the word we are trying to say. But these jokes hide our fears that we will be one of those members of the population who truly do suffer from senility and Alzheimer's. There are many other reasons we may be forgetful. Increased stress can keep our minds occupied. Vitamin deficiencies, cardiovascular disease, simple disuse of brain cells, and other factors must be eliminated as legitimate causes of forgetfulness and memory impairment. After all other possible causes of memory reduction have been eliminated, then we need to consider Alzheimer's disease as a possibility. Many studies also indicate that mental "fuzziness" resulting from lack of sleep, poor nutrition, lack of exercise, or simple disuse of those neuronal connections can be misinterpreted as the beginnings of Alzheimer's disease. Don't live in fear that the doctor may tell you something you don't want to hear. Your doctor may tell you that you suffer from a simple vitamin deficiency and that changes to your diet will take care of the problem.

One other possibility for memory impairment in women is a lack of estrogen. Women in their thirties who had certain diseases and were receiving estrogen-suppressing drugs exhibit verbal, but not visual or spatial, memory loss and reduced levels of concentration. Men also have estrogen receptors in their brains. Researchers are beginning to examine the possibility that estrogen therapy may improve memory function in men as well. You need to weigh the risks against the benefits. *Estrogen replacement therapy* (ERT), although proven to be effective in reducing the symptoms of senility and Alzheimer's disease in women, is not for everyone. Although ERT helps control osteoporosis, improves memory, improves coordination, and protects against Alzheimer's, it also is thought to increase

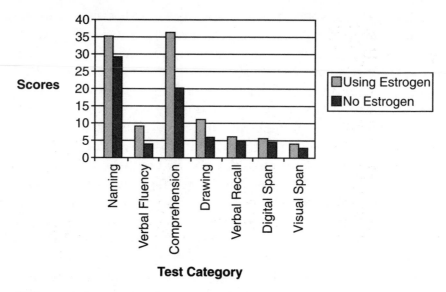

Figure 6-5 Test Scores for Women Alzheimer's Patients. Data from Jon Queijo, "Tracking the Estrogen Effect, Connections to Memory and Alzheimer's Disease," *Brain Work* (January/February, 1998): 1-3.

the risk of endometrial and breast cancer. For women with a family history of breast cancer, ERT may not be an appropriate therapy. Consult your doctor.

Notice the test scores for women diagnosed with Alzheimer's disease who were and were not using estrogen therapy. In all cases, the women using estrogen scored higher, especially on comprehension tests.

Notice Figure 6-6, which demonstrates the results of estrogen therapy on a group of retired women. This study demonstrates that those who took estrogen longer had a significantly lower risk of Alzheimer's disease.

Nonsteroidal anti-inflammatory medications such as Ibuprofen actually may reduce the risk of Alzheimer's. People who had taken these drugs for a minimum of two years had half the risk of Alzheimer's disease as those who had not taken the drug.[22]

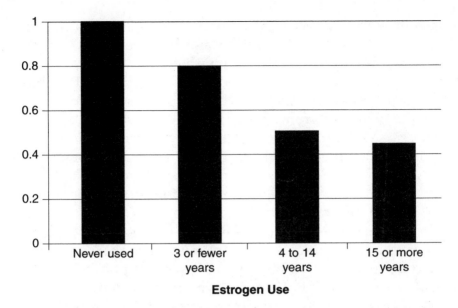

Figure 6-6 Relative Risk of Contracting Alzheimer's Disease. Data from Jon Queijo, "Tracking the Estrogen Effect, Connections to Memory and Alzheimer's Disease," *Brain Work* (January/February, 1998): 1-3.

Vitamin E and ginkgo, rich in antioxidants, also have been demonstrated to slow the progress of Alzheimer's disease in more than half the patients taking these supplements. Ginkgo is a regulated drug in Europe. In the 1980s, it was the drug most widely prescribed, at 120 mg daily, to increase concentration. The standard dosage was 40 mg, with 24 percent ginkgo flavoneglycosides and 6 percent terpenelactone as the active ingredients, taken three times daily. Although this dose of ginkgo is considered safe, it has a mild blood-thinning effect and can lead to restlessness, diarrhea, or vomiting in some users. Vitamin E was given at a dose of 2,000 I.U. per day, and studies indicate that it increased the amount of time before Alzheimer's patients required institutional care. Note that 800 I.U. per day of vitamin E is considered safe and that increasing the dose to 2,000 I.U. per day can increase the risk of bleeding.[23] Antioxidants reduce the damage caused by free radicals and have been linked to reducing the risk of cognitive impairment.

The effects of vitamin and herbal supplements sometimes are controversial. It is possible to overdose and harm yourself. Recall from earlier discussions that you must check with your doctor first before you embark into new self-help territory, especially if you already are taking some medications.

Some researchers believe that having a high degree of education and maintaining a high level of mental activity protect the brain against the ravaging effects of Alzheimer's. Learning new things keeps the brain's connections robust and flourishing. This gives you a greater supply of connections to use as surplus in order to maintain your mental ability if Alzheimer's disease does affect you.

Doctors and Medication

We cannot begin to impress on you enough the importance of a yearly physical exam. As you can tell from the information we have presented regarding sleep, nutrition, exercise, psychological attitude, and spiritual values, your mental health and physical health are intimately intertwined. Sometimes what we think are irreparable consequences of aging can be corrected. If you notice changes, especially if they are sudden, in memory, energy levels, or even just a general feeling that all is not well, seek out your doctor. Have your doctor test you for inappropriate hormonal levels, vitamin deficiencies, high blood pressure, and so on. And if you check out fine and are physically able to start an exercise program, try various techniques described in the text to get those muscles moving and oxygen pumping.

If your doctor cannot find anything wrong with you, but you still do not feel quite right, get a second or even third opinion. For example, Virginia Chestnut (whom you met earlier) suffered for many years from high blood pressure that was not adequately controlled by medications. She also felt "bone-tired" all the time and would fall asleep within minutes of sitting down. Three doctors, including a geriatric specialist, did not find an underlying condition that might cause the symptoms and just prescribed more medication. After all, she thought, she wasn't 29 anymore. Within 10 minutes of meeting her, a cardiologist using only a stethoscope determined that both carotid arteries (which feed the brain) and the arteries to her kidneys (which elevated the blood pressure) probably were blocked. Further testing confirmed his diagnosis. Surgeries to remove the blockages reduced Virginia's blood pressure and improved her memory, and she no longer falls asleep whenever she sits down. That was two years ago when she was 79. She is now 81, and a stronger, more vigorous woman you will never meet.

We tell you this story to illustrate our assertion that you know your body. You've lived in it your whole life. If you don't feel your doctor is meeting your needs, find another one. It only takes one right opinion to start you on the road to better health, happier spirits, and clearer thoughts.

Now let's address medications. Many medications slow the brain. Simple over-the-counter antihistamines come with the warning not to operate heavy machinery while taking the medicine. That's because it slows the speed of your mental processing and reaction time. Heavy machinery, by the way, includes your car and the riding lawn mower. Other medication, as previously mentioned, can disrupt your sleep patterns, dull the senses with which you input information, or affect your nutritional intake.

Read the labels. Become a more careful consumer of your medications. Check with your pharmacist and doctor for side effects. Perhaps, if you feel like your brain is packed in cotton or are experiencing other side affects, you can switch medications. Another consideration is medicinal interactions. My husband, for example, who has had a severe heart attack, takes numerous medications. The doctor and pharmacist were keeping an eye on everything, and the pharmacist's computer was programmed to flag for various interactions (including this particular one). But things sometimes slip through the system, and it wasn't until two of my husband's medications ran out at the same time that the pharmacist saw the two prescriptions together and immediately informed us that we needed to contact the doctor.

Take *all* of your medications to your doctor *and* to the pharmacist. Ask the pharmacist to check them all and determine whether there are any potential adverse interactions. And when you are doing this, bring along your vitamins and supplements.

CONCLUSION

We hope that you have learned a few facts in this chapter that you did not know and found a few ideas to integrate into your lifestyle. Because rehearsals are one of the learning techniques you are incorporating and practicing, let's take a minute to recap.

Research has identified many factors associated with successful aging and maintenance of mental agility. Briefly discussing each one, let's start with your general health. The absence of diseases and good overall health indicate that your body is performing at an adequate level and is able to provide the support (nutritional and physical) that your brain requires to operate efficiently. Another factor was high socioeconomic status. Having a little extra access to other members of society and having at least a little money for extras allows you to indulge yourself in more educational activities and the stimulating environment that is conducive to mental animation. But if you do not have a lot of money, there are plenty of free opportunities for exercising those mental muscles. Visiting the library, having a friend over to your house, and going to rehearsals of plays and musical performances are all possibilities for exercising your mind. A stimulating environment keeps those neurons popping and creates new connections. Search out new interests and new opportunities. Many colleges will let seniors take classes at a reduced rate or will waive the fees entirely (see Appendix A). Next, having a flexible personality is an indication that you are willing to try new things. And last, but not least, keep in contact with your friends. Practice those mental skills. Have little contests to see who has the better memory. The loser has to practice harder the next week.

SELF-QUIZ

Here is a self-assessment on the six characteristics associated with successful aging and mental agility. For each one, list what you now are working on for developing these characteristics and then identify three things in each characteristic that you can start doing to regain your brain.

What am I doing now for my brain?	**What can I start doing to regain my brain?**

Absence of cardiovascular and other diseases

1. _____ 1. _____
2. _____ 2. _____
3. _____ 3. _____

High socioeconomic status

1. _____ 1. _____
2. _____ 2. _____
3. _____ 3. _____

Involvement in a complex and intellectually stimulating environment

1. _____ 1. _____
2. _____ 2. _____
3. _____ 3. _____

Flexible personality at midlife

1. _____ 1. _____
2. _____ 2. _____
3. _____ 3. _____

High cognitive status of spouse

1. _____ 1. _____
2. _____ 2. _____
3. _____ 3. _____

Maintenance of high levels of perceptual processing speed

1. _____ 1. _____
2. _____ 2. _____
3. _____ 3. _____

In the next chapter, we are going to provide you with many, many games and activities to promote a strong, active, efficient mind and memory. Keep in mind, however, that as you learn something and become comfortable with that idea or technique, you need to move on into unexplored territory. Recall Figure 4-1, where a PET scan demonstrated the different areas of the brain that are activated for a verbal skill when it is new and when it is practiced. You need to keep trying new things. If you like to work jigsaw puzzles and you are very fast at it, move on up to 3D puzzles. If you have found great success with rehearsal strategies, begin to include listmaking or visualization strategies.

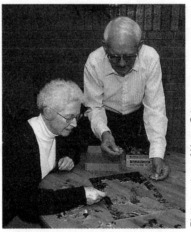

Photo courtesy of Henry Ortega

Older and Wiser

Helen and Gene McLane, married for almost 50 years, still love to play games together. Jigsaw puzzles, 3-D puzzles, and crossword puzzles are some of their favorite activities. They have also been know to race each other for the best times and scores on their new computer. They are two of the most physically and mentally active people we know..

Start looking for opportunities to apply these lifestyles. Share the ideas with your friends. Get a buddy to brainstorm with for new things to do and try. You can do this. Just start with one new thing you want to alter, master that, and then incorporate another lifestyle change. In our household, it was always the joke that as my father aged, he asked us to just put him in the corner with a wooden bowl. You have a choice: independent living or relegation to the corner with a wooden bowl.

REFERENCES:

1. Lynne Lamberg, "A Matter of Time," BrainWork (March–April 1998): 6–8.
2. Isadora Stehlin, "A Time to Heal: Chronotherapy Tunes In to Body's Rhythms," FDA Consumer, 31 (April 1, 1997).
3. Avi Karni et al., "Dependence on REM sleep of overnight improvement of a perceptual skill," Science, 265 (July 29, 1994): 679–682.
4. Matthew Wilson and Bruce McNaughton cited in "Memory Building," The Economist, 348 (August 29, 1998).
5. Timothy Monk et al., "Subjective alertness rhythms in elderly people," Journal of Biological Rhythms (September 1996): 208–276.
6. George Nobbe, "Resetting internal clocks," Omni (January 1995).
7. D. Garfinkel et al., "Improvement of sleep quality in elderly people by controlled-release melatonin," Lancet (August 26, 1995): 541–544.
8. Sonia Ancoli-Israel, "Sleep problems in older adults: putting myths to bed," Geriatrics, 52 (January 1, 1997): 20–26.
9. Anonymous, "The sleep cure for memory lapses," HEALTH (March 1997).
10. Sonia Ancoli-Israel, "Sleep problems in older adults: putting myths to bed,"

11. Mike Snider, "Tennis and the Brain," Tennis USTA (October, 1996): 9–11.
12. Eus J.W. Van Someren et al., "Long-term fitness training improves the circadian rest-activity rhythm in healthy elderly males," Journal of Biological Rhythms (April 1997): 146–156.
13. Jet (March 9, 1998): 24.
14. Donald T. Kirkendall and William E. Garrett, Jr., "The effects of aging and training on skeletal muscle," American Journal of Sports Medicine, 26(4): 598–602.
15. The 1998 Health Guide, Baltimore County Department of Aging (Baltimore County, Maryland, 1998).
16. Roy J. Shephard, Aging, Physical Activity and Health (Champaign, IL: Human Kinetics, 1997).
17. Doralie Denenberg Segal, Carlos J. Crespo, and Ellen Smit, "Active Seniors: Protect them, don't neglect them," Public Health Reports, 113 (2): 137–139.
18. Renee Solomon, "Coping with Stress: A physician's guide to mental health in aging," Geriatrics (July 1996): 46–52.
19. David Mahoney and Richard Restak, "The Longevity Strategy. How to Live to 100 using the Brain-Body Connection," BrainWork (March–April 1998): 1–5.
20. Robert Sapolsky, Stress, the Aging Brain, and the Mechanisms of Neuron Death (MIT Press, 1992).
21. Dr. Robert Goldman, "Mind over Matter: Anti-stress tips for anti-aging," Total Health (July 1997): 26–27.
22. Diana Sugg, "Drug's Bonus Effect Weighed," The Baltimore Sun (March 10, 1997): 1A.
23. No author noted, "Staving off Senility," Harvard Women's Health Watch (December 1997).

C h a p t e r

7

Enjoy Your Ageless Mental Agility

Game Your Way to Ageless Mental Agility

KEY CONCEPTS

Schaie's Results—The Big Payoff
Strategies to Improve Mental Ability
Mental Agility Pretest
Mental Agility Exercises
Mental Agility Posttest
Mental Development Activities

INTRODUCTION

> *"It is not how old you are, but how you are old."—*
> *Marie Dressler*

So after all this, what do we really mean by Ageless Mental Agility? *Ageless* summons up a vision of freedom from chronological constraints. *Mental* sounds like the perfect blend of brain and mind. *Agility* feels like an ability to freely respond in novel ways to solve new problems. Let's examine why this book culminates in this final burst of energy.

In Chapter 6, you learned about the results of various studies that demonstrated a relationship between your health and your mental agility. Also, remember (of course you do—you've been practicing) that in Chapter 2 we showed you the various areas of the brain. We discussed them in reference to Gardner's multiple intelligences, which are linguistic, musical, logical-mathematical, spatial, kinesthetic, naturalist, and personal. Like a body builder who wants the entire physique well developed and strong, you want all aspects of your mental abilities to be vigorous and well developed. Chapter 6 dealt with many of these intelligences in the context of possible alterations and improvements to your way of life.

We have given you many suggestions on methods to improve the quality of your life throughout this text and discussed why each one was important to both your overall health and your mental agility. These suggested strategies were based on well-grounded research by many individuals and groups. One of the researchers we mentioned was Dr. K. Warner Schaie. We are going to introduce you to some of his other results and especially those he obtained working with Dr. Sherry Willis, his wife. If you have been skimming over the technical sections of the book so far, we encourage you to read this section anyway. This is the basis of our reasons for writing this book. This is, shall we say, The Big Payoff.

THE BIG PAYOFF

K. Warner Schaie directs one of the most extensive longitudinal research programs on intellectual functions over the adult ages. The Seattle Longitudinal Study began in 1956. More than 5,000 participants ranging in age from 22 to 95 were interviewed and tested in seven-year cycles. Results indicated that participants gained in proficiency through their early forties and then functioned at approximately the same level throughout the rest of their forties through their late fifties or sixties. As Table 7-1 indicates, most participants actually maintained stable performances on most cognitive

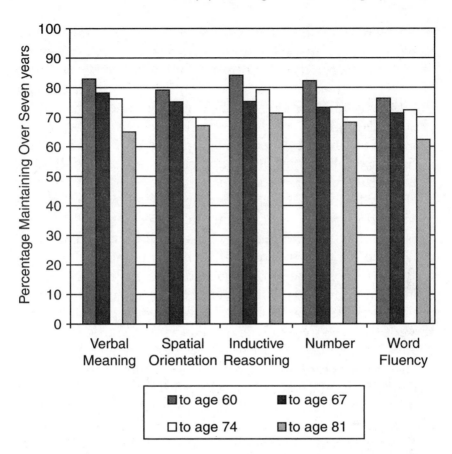

Table 7-1 Proportion of Individuals Who Maintain Stable Levels of Performance Over Seven Years on Primary Abilities, Schaie, 1996.

abilities well into old age. As late as their sixties, most people do not show significant changes in mental abilities from the last testing. By their eighties, most people have experienced some decline in at least one area. Moreover, between the ages of 74 and 81, less than half showed mental declines on all of the mental activities tested. The other half showed declines in some but not all abilities, particularly those requiring psychomotor speed.

Other studies, such as the Baltimore Longitudinal Study of Aging (BLSA), confirm these results. The BLSA has followed more than 2,000 participants since 1958. Results indicate that as we age past our sixties, our ability to remember figures and shapes may decrease, but our vocabulary increases into our eighties and then may decrease slightly.[1] This increase in our vocabulary skills is thought to be due to use and increased exposure throughout our life to words. As we age, however, many of us are not called on to practice and exercise skills such as spatial abilities, logic, and so on, and so it is thought that these skills decrease due to disuse.

Dr. Willis and Dr. Schaie wanted to determine whether modest declines in specific mental processes could be reversed in healthy individuals. This would lend greater credence to the theory that mental declines in otherwise healthy individuals could be attributed to disuse. A Primary Mental Ability Test had been administered to the subjects participating in the Seattle Longitudinal Study 14 years prior to this intervention strategy and was used as a benchmark. From this group, 229 subjects from 64 to 75 years old and in good health, who exhibited marked losses in mental functioning over the past 14 years, were selected to determine whether mental performances could be improved through tutoring and practice of skills. Dr. Schaie and Dr. Willis embarked on a training program to improve mental functioning in a set of the participants. These participants were given five one-hour sessions aimed at improving basic abilities such as inductive reasoning and spatial abilities and offered strategies for tackling tasks such as memorization. The seniors then were tested again. Their results were stunning.

After merely five one-hour training sessions, 66 percent of the seniors improved dramatically and 40 percent regained up to 14 years in mental ability.

Approximately 66 percent demonstrated significant improvement. Some 40 percent regained everything they had lost over the years, scoring as well or better than they had 14 years earlier. Still more stunning is that this advance persisted for at least seven more years without further training."[2] When checked on seven years later, they still demon-strated a distinct advantage compared to those who had not received the training.

After seven years, without further training, these se-niors maintained this improvement.

You may recall from earlier chapters that how much you, as an individual, decline is dependent on many things, such as genetics, disease, level of activity, and so on. Some of these factors, such as genetics, you obviously cannot change. K. Warner Schaie identified six of the factors associ-ated with retaining strong mental functions that you may be able to control:

1. Absence of cardiovascular and other diseases
2. High socioeconomic status
3. Involvement in complex and intellectually stimulating environment
4. Flexible personality at midlife
5. High cognitive status of spouse
6. Maintenance of high levels of perceptual processing speed

In Chapter 6, we talked about how to control the first five factors in the list. We are going to discuss number 6 and readdress numbers 3 and 4 in this chapter within the context of training, exercising, and rejuvenating those brain cells.

In this chapter, you will have an opportunity to take a preassessment test, experience a set of training exercises, and then retest to assess your gains.

In general, to combat the effects of cognitive decline, you can

1. **Accommodate:** You alter the activities you used to per-form. You may start to write things down to help you re-member ideas that you are reading about.
2. **Compensate:** Use additional processes to supplement your abilities and maintain your usual activities. You

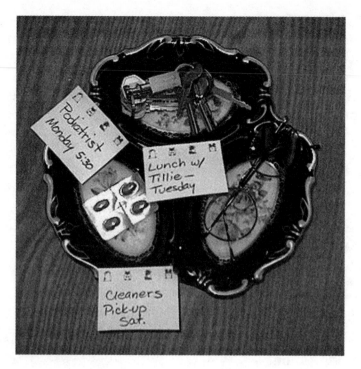

Figure 7-1 The Ugly Plate

may use glasses to allow you to read as comfortably as before or select the large-print editions.

3. **Remediate:** Intervene by improving the affected ability. Investigate eye surgery to fix the problem once and for all.

We have focused on compensation strategies and remediation strategies in this text. One of the methods you can use to compensate is external memory aids. One of the more interesting research studies involved the use of an ugly plate as a visual mnemonic device for seniors to use as a memory aid (see Figure 7-1). The plate was a cheap plastic three-section picnic plate in the ugliest color the researchers could find. The plate was placed in a prominent place in the home (where you couldn't possibly miss it). It could only be removed for social occasions. Items to be remembered, such as glasses or medicines, were placed on the plate. Sticky notes (in a contrasting color) with terse, one-line descriptions of a specific activity that needed to be done, were placed at odd angles on the rim of the plate. This device, which could be vividly recalled as needed, reduced the frequency of every-day memory lapses an average of 57 percent to 65 percent.[3] What a wonderful idea and so simple and inexpensive an approach. Just remember that we are going for visually memorable, and the more obnoxious the color combination, the better.

Here are a few other strategies:

- Make a list.
- Place frequently needed objects in the same place.
- Leave yourself notes.
- Twist your watch around on your wrist so that every occasion you check for the time and have to turn the watch, you can rehearse what you are trying to remember.

Now we want to give you the chance we promised you to test your cognitive abilities, learn some remediation strate-gies, practice them, and test your cognitive abilities again. Before you start, though, we want to remind you of a few things.

- You tested yourself already to determine whether you are an auditory, visual, or kinesthetic learner. While try-ing to incorporate the mental exercises and techniques that follow, try to use your preferred method of re-hearsal. Also, include the other techniques as much as possible, even if they are not your preferred method. You want all of those areas recording information, and the more modes of inputting information you use, the more you should recall.
- Similar memories may be confusing due to the number of associations in your mind. Try to find the differences among the various techniques as well as the similarities.

For example, can you remember the details of the last time you went to the bank? You probably can remember going to a grandchild's recital, however. Unique situations stick in your mind, while many instances of the same situation may run together.

- If you are practicing one of the techniques or completing an exercise, distractions may make you forget where you were. So if you get lost in the middle of an exercise, perhaps you should find a good starting point and go again. Try to notice whether you lose track of what you're doing with or without distractions.

- Some information never makes it to long-term memory. Not paying adequate attention accounts for approximately 50 percent of reported memory problems. Concentrate on what you want to remember. Try to make associations and use some of the techniques previously discussed. The inability to rapidly form associations is what accounts for much of the effect of aging on measured cognitive abilities. If you need to remember something you need to do, concentrate and come up with little sayings or rhymes, or even write it down so that it will make more associations. The more you associate new information with items already firmly entrenched in your memory, the more likely you will be able to recall the new information successfully.

- One of the most common complaints by the elderly (and the young) is the increasing inability to recall names and particular words. The *tip-of-the-tongue* (TOT) phenomenon is when individuals *know* that they know the name but cannot recall it at that particular moment. Ninety-two percent of the time, when older adults say they know a name but just cannot immediately recall it, they are correct. They actually do know it. Therefore, when people say they know something, believe them. One research study demonstrated a 48 percent retrieval success rate within two to three minutes without any external aids.

These were the strategies used for successful retrieval in the study previously described:

- 27 percent use an alphabet strategy. (I know it starts with a "b.")
- 10 percent use a visualization strategy. (Where was the last time I saw those?)
- 26 percent use an association strategy. (Let's see, I know that he works with Janet . . .)
- 37 percent use a pop-into-the-head (in a blinding flash of light) strategy.[4]

So if you just *know* you have the answer to the exercises and games, try one of the strategies just mentioned and give yourself two to three minutes to locate and retrieve the needed information before you give up on yourself.

Are any of these strategies and techniques new? Are you learning a new skill? In the beginning, it is hard to remember details (such as how to decide what the next number in a series is), but with more repetition and experience, you can create more associations and remember strategies easily and efficiently.

Does it take longer to learn? It may while you are integrating new techniques. Don't be discouraged. Keep these tips in mind:

- **Be aware.** Now you know you may have to work harder.
- **Pay attention.** Concentrate on what you really want to remember.
- **Associate.** Associate what you want to know with what you already know.
- **Practice remembering.** Choose a technique and try it out.

Do you recall Gardner's multiple intelligences presented in Chapter 2? We used them to identify the various areas of the brain that perform different types of functions. Now here are some brief suggestions for activities to stimulate those areas of the brain. Try to incorporate as many as you can to exercise multiple areas of your brain. Choose one or two to start. Set a goal and get started. Generate as many mental connections as you can.

 Spatial Intelligence

- Do jigsaw puzzles.
- Do 3D puzzles.
- Build a house of cards.
- Build model cars.
- Fly model airplanes (or sail boats).
- Arrange flowers.
- Paint.
- Do ceramics.
- Play charades.

 Musical Intelligence

- Develop an interest in classical music.
- Make up jingles to remember things.
- Whistle, hum, or sing.
- Learn to play the instrument you always wanted to learn when you were younger.

 Math/Logical Intelligence

- Get puzzle books.
- Balance your checkbook by hand instead of using a computer.
- Do brain teasers.

- Solve mazes.
- Play bridge or other card games.

Linguistic Intelligence

- Do crossword puzzles.
- Join a club associated with your hobby.
- Write down your memories or the memories of your ancestors, or dictate them into a recorder.
- Invite friends over for dinner and play board games (the more the board games require you to talk, the better).
- Play Scrabble™ or Scribbage™ or Password™ or Boggle™.

Kinesthetic Intelligence

- Turn on the radio and dance around the house.
- Exercise in a class or with a tape.
- Take an advanced exercise class.
- Learn tai chi.
- Take up a hobby that requires detailed use of the hands, such as needlepoint.
- Make a tall-ships model.
- Play charades.

Personal Intelligence

- Join a club.
- Volunteer at a local school.
- Write a family history.
- Plan a family reunion.
- Keep a diary.
- Plan a self-improvement program.

- Make a list of the 10 most important events in your life.
- Make a list of the 10 most important things in your life.
- Make a list of the 10 most important people in your life.
- Work for a charitable cause.
- Take a pie to a neighbor, and sit and chat a while.
- Visit someone in the hospital.
- Write a card to someone who is lonely.

Continuing-education courses, crossword puzzles, or anything that uses your brainpower could be beneficial. "Play bridge instead of bingo." According to Dr. Schaie, "The only negative we found was bingo, unless maybe you play 20 cards at once."[5]

So as you go through these training exercises for your mind, relax, look for associations, and try to incorporate the various learning strategies presented in Chapter 4. Dust off those neuron connections, and let's get going!

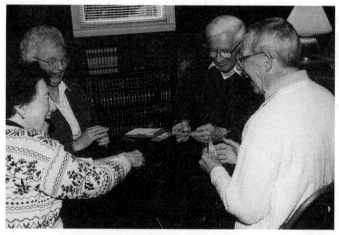

The Giffords and the Austins share a joke over the bridge table.

Photo courtesy of Winfield Leitzer

MENTAL AGILITY PRETEST

 The results of the following test will not yield an *intelligence quotient* (IQ) rating. If you would like to have a measure of your IQ, several Web sites will provide this for you. You might try www.intp.org/tests.html, which offers, in their words, "a plethora of tests." This pretest will provide a raw score against which you may compare your posttest score.

Find some scratch paper for use during the test. Set a timer for 10 minutes. Begin the test, and mark answers for each question in the space provided.

BEGIN

In each of the following items, write the correct number or letter of the picture that completes the pattern.

Exercise 7-1a

_____ 1. B D F H **?**

_____ 2.

_____ 3.

_____ 4. 30, 29, 27, 24, 20, **?**

_____ 5.

_____ 6.

_____ 7.

_____ 8.

_____ 9. 1, 6, 16, 21, 31, **?**

_____ 10.

_____ 11.

_____ 12.

_____ 13.

_____ 14. 1, 3, 9, 27, **?**

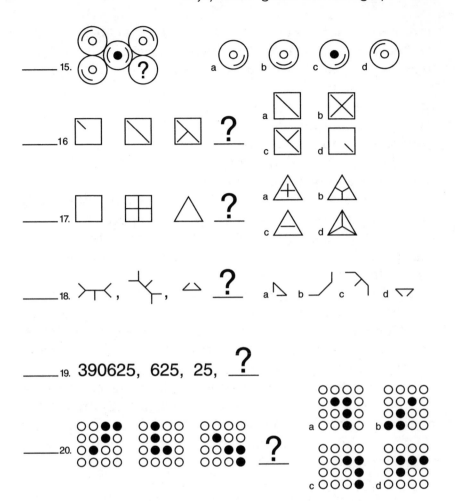

_____ 15.

_____ 16

_____ 17.

_____ 18.

_____ 19. 390625, 625, 25, **?**

_____ 20.

After the 10 minutes have elapsed, check your answers at the end of this chapter in the "Answers" section. Record the number correct. After you have a chance to practice inductive-reasoning and spatial-relationship skills, take the posttest at the end of this chapter.

MENTAL AGILITY EXERCISES

Inductive Reasoning

One of the key questions regarding intelligence or high mental ability is whether a person can recognize patterns and predict the next item in a pattern. This is called *inductive reasoning*. To a large extent, inductive reasoning is a learned skill. For the most difficult problems, however, insight and creativity are needed—two qualities that are considered to be possessed by very intelligent people. On the Mental Ability Pretest, the questions that ask for the next item in a sequence are inductive-reasoning problems.

A large portion of inductive-reasoning problems involves numbers, and a word of caution is required here. It is not uncommon for people to slide over numbers while they are reading. Numbers are not perceived to be important for some people. In fact, they think the numbers are superfluous, interrupt their reading, and get in the way of the meaning of the sentences. If you consider yourself a number skipper, you might think about developing a facility for observing and incorporating numbers into the text you read. Some people are fond of saying, "Oh, I've never been very good at math." Well, here is your chance to get good at math. There is a saying in mathematics that "a mathematician is a pattern seeker." The following section will help you develop pattern-seeking skills.

You can employ several strategies to determine a numerical pattern from a sequence of numbers. The place to start is identifying the pattern. In the following sequence, you can predict the next number:

1,2,3,4,5,6, . . .

The next number is, of course, 7. You knew that. What you may not realize is that you recognized the pattern as the counting numbers and retrieved the seven from long-term memory. There are so many connections to this pattern of numbers that you probably were not aware of the recall mechanism at work! This process of immediate recall is quite different from problem solving. In problem solving, you do not have the answer already stored in memory. You must identify the question, note all of the facts you already have, and then determine what is missing. After you figure out what is missing, the creative work begins. We will apply this sequence of steps to a few inductive-reasoning numerical problems.

Find the next term in this sequence:
5, 10, 15, 20, . . .

To solve this problem, you would go through these steps:

1. **Identify the question.** You need to find the next number in the sequence.

2. **Note all of the facts you already have.** You have four terms already. They appear to be a collection of 1s, 5s, and 0s, with one 2.

3. **Determine what is missing.** You don't know the pattern. (You may know already, but it will help to follow the sequence of inductive-reasoning steps to learn the process).

4. **Do some creative work.** Take a look at how each term is built from the ones before it.

Notice that the numbers go up by 5 each time. This is the five times table. You have $1 \times 5, 2 \times 5, 3 \times 5$, and 4×5. Predict that the next term is $5 \times 5 = 25$.

Find the next term in this sequence:
1, 1, 2, 3, 5, 8, 13, . . .

Follow these steps:

1. **Identify the question.** You need to find the next number in the sequence.

2. **Note all of the facts you already have.** You have seven terms already. Except for the second term, they increase in value. The increase is not the same.

3. **Determine what is missing.** You don't know the pattern.

4. **Do some creative work.** Take a look at how each term is built from the one before it.

Notice that $1 + 1 = 2, 1 + 2 = 3, 2 + 3 = 5, 3 + 5 = 8$, and $5 + 8 = 13$. Each number after the first two is the sum of the two numbers before it. Predict that $8 + 13 = 21$ is the next term in the sequence. This is a famous sequence called the *Fibonacci sequence,* named after the Italian mathematician who studied it. For a more in-depth treatment of the sequence, visit the Web site www.mathacademy.com/platonic_realms/en-cyclop/articles/fibonac.html.

This next sequence takes you up a notch on the difficulty scale! Find the next term in this sequence:

1,101,1101,101101, . . .

Follow these steps:

1. **Identify the question.** You need to find the next number in the sequence.

2. **Note all of the facts you already have.** You have four terms already. They appear to be a collection of 1s and 0s.

3. **Determine what is missing.** You don't know the pattern.

4. **Do some creative work.** Take a look at how each term is built from the terms before it.

Notice from 1 to 101, it looks as if you put a 10 in front of the 1 to make the second term.	1, 101,
But you didn't do that for the third term. You put a 1 in front of the second term.	1, 101, 1101,
Notice the fourth term. Here you are back to putting a 10 in front.	1, 101, 1101, 101101
So, now you guess that you put a 1 in front of the fourth term to make the fifth term.	1, 101, 1101, 101101, 1101101

Notice that the word is *guess*. That's the best you can do for inductive reasoning. Whatever pattern you make up, someone else might devise a different pattern.

Here are a few other common strategies for finding the next number in a sequence. Consider the sequence 1, 3, 5, 7, 9, 11, 13, . . . What is the next number in the sequence? You might recognize the sequence as a list of the odd numbers. Then next number would be 15. If you didn't recognize the odd numbers, you might try looking for a pattern. You would see that the numbers go up by 2 each time. So the next number would be $13 + 2 = 15$.

Consider this sequence: 1, 4, 9, 16, 25, . . . What is the next number in the sequence? You might recognize that this is a sequence of perfect squares.

The first term is $1 \times 1 = 1$.
The second term is $2 \times 2 = 4$.
The third term is $3 \times 3 = 9$.
The fourth term is $4 \times 4 = 16$.
The fifth term is $5 \times 5 = 25$.

Predict that the pattern would continue, and the sixth term would be $6 \times 6 = 36$.

Consider this sequence: 1, 3, 6, 10, . . .
Follow these steps:

1. **Identify the question.** You need to find the next number in the sequence.

2. **Note all of the facts you already have.** You have four terms already. They appear to be getting larger. They are not consecutive numbers. They are not the perfect squares.

3. **Determine what is missing.** You don't know the pattern.

4. **Do some creative work.** Take a look at how each term is built from the one before it.

You might add $1 + 2$ to get to 3, but $3 + 2$ is not 6. $3 + 3$ is 6. What do you add to 6 to get to 10? Well, it's 4. Write the numbers in a table, and take a look at the pattern.

$$1$$
$$1 + 2 = 3$$
$$3 + 3 = 6$$
$$6 + 4 = 10$$

Now you can see the pattern. Each time, you add the next counting number to the term. Often a visual aid such as creating a table helps you identify a pattern you may not notice in paragraph form.

To help build spatial-relationship skills, view these numbers in a picture.

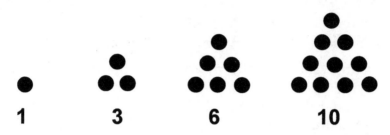

The triangular arrangement prompts us to name this sequence the *triangular numbers*. Looking at the pattern of dots, decide how adding a counting number each time adds dots to the figures.

The next exercise requires that you perform long division. You may prefer to use a calculator, but the display may not hold enough digits for you to recognize the pattern. Complete the following table and then look for patterns. Notice that the division will never end, so stop after 12 digits in your answers. As soon as you recognize the pattern, test one more number, and then fill in the Quotient block from the pattern. Answers are at the end of this chapter.

Division	Quotient
$1 \div 7$	0._ _ _ _ _ _ _ _ _ _ _ _
$2 \div 7$	0._ _ _ _ _ _ _ _ _ _ _ _
$3 \div 7$	0._ _ _ _ _ _ _ _ _ _ _ _
$4 \div 7$	0._ _ _ _ _ _ _ _ _ _ _ _
$5 \div 7$	0._ _ _ _ _ _ _ _ _ _ _ _
$6 \div 7$	0._ _ _ _ _ _ _ _ _ _ _ _

Notice the patterns within the quotients that relate to 7? Examine the Quotient column. Do you see that there is a 14 and 28 in each number? That is 2×7 and 4×7. Another pattern is that the first digits in the quotients are in ascending order. If you remember the sequence of numbers in the repeating section, then you can dazzle your friends and confound your enemies with math magic tricks and lightning-speed division prowess!

Not all sequences involve numbers. Consider this sequence of letters:

S, M, T, W, T, F, S

They are the first letters of the days of the week. What do you think the next letter is in the following sequence of letters?

O, T, T, F, F, S, S, E, N, . . .

These are the first letters of the words for the counting numbers, 1, 2, 3, 4, 5, 6, 7, 8, 9, . . .

Sequence of Letters

Here's another: A, E, F, H, . . . What is the next letter in this sequence? _____ The answer is at the end of this chapter.

This sequence is another favorite for building pattern-recognition powers. In the blanks in the table, write the counting numbers down the first column and then up the second column. Do this before you go on to the next paragraph.

Take some time to study the list of numbers that you generated. What do you recognize about the list of numbers? Do this before you go on to the next paragraph.

$$
\begin{array}{cc}
1 & 8 \\
2 & \underline{\hphantom{0}} \\
\underline{\hphantom{0}} & \underline{\hphantom{0}} \\
\underline{\hphantom{0}} & \underline{\hphantom{0}} \\
\underline{\hphantom{0}} & \underline{\hphantom{0}} \\
\underline{\hphantom{0}} & 2 \\
\underline{\hphantom{0}} & 1 \\
\underline{\hphantom{0}} & 0 \\
\end{array}
$$

Did you recognize this as the nine times table? The pattern that is generated by the nine times table yields great fun. Try this: Add the digits across each row in the table. For example, for the row containing 18, add 1 + 8. Then 2 + 7, and so on.

You found another pattern. The sum is always 9. Here is the fun part. Because the numbers always add up to 9, you only need nine fingers to represent the numbers in the table. You can use your hands to multiply by 9. Consider the diagram in Figure 7-2. Place your hands on the table in the same manner.

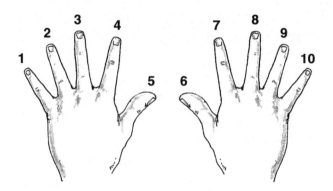

Figure 7-2 Number assigned to digits

Suppose you want to show **4 x 9.** Tuck the finger numbered **4,** the index finger of your left hand, under your hand. This may be difficult at first if you have arthritis in your hands, but the exercise may improve your flexibility! There are **3** fingers up on the left of finger **#4,** and there are **6** to the right. **3, 6:** The answer to **4 x 9** is **36.** See Figure 7-3.

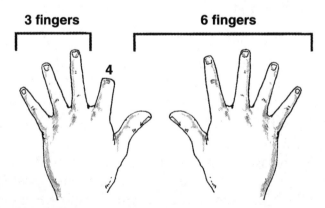

Figure 7-3 4 times 9 is 36

Try this again. This time you'll multiply **6 x 9**. First tuck finger **#6**, the thumb of your right hand, under your hand, as in Figure 7-4. There are **5** fingers up on the left of finger number **6** and **4** fingers up on the right of finger number **6** **Six times nine is 54.**

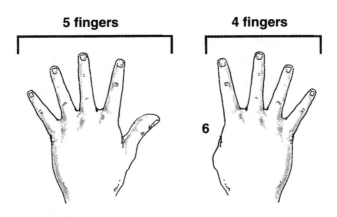

5 fingers   **4 fingers**

6

Figure 7-4   6 times 9 is 54

This is something you might share with someone else. Practice a few times by yourself, and then teach this trick to a friend or a child who is learning the multiplication tables.

 Inductive Reasoning Exercises

In each problem, write the next term in the sequence. Also, write the reason why you think that is the next term.

1. 1, 5, 9, 13, . . .   _____ _____

2. D, H, L, . . .   _____ _____

3. 15, 14, 12, 9, . . .   _____ _____

4. 1, 10, 3, 12, 5, 14, 7, . . .   _____ _____

5. 625, 125, 25, . . .   _____ _____

6. J, F, M, A, M, . . .   _____ _____

7. 1, 8, 27, 64, . . .   _____ _____

8. 1, 101, 1001, 10001, . . .   _____ _____

9. B, C, D, G, J, . . .   _____ _____

10. Q, W, E, R, T, . . .   _____ _____

SPATIAL RELATIONSHIPS

 Knowing where you are with respect to other objects, distinguishing between two similar objects, and finding similarities between two objects are examples of skills in *spatial relationships*. In general, having good spatial-relationship skills means that you are comfortable and working well with the three-dimensional world. Kinesthetic learners usually have wonderful spatial-relationship skills. They seldom get lost. They know where their keys are! They function well with their bodies. Often, they are fine athletes. They make fine quilters. They generally possess the body/kinesthetic intelligence Gardner tells us about. Those of us without a native ability in this area require training to develop spatial-relationship skills. This section provides an introduction to and exercises in *spatial relationships* (SR).

First, consider inductive reasoning with objects. This will carry over from the previous section and tie in spatial skills. You will use a table of objects as your "space." Each section of your table contains a special character, a ✳. If you would like to name this object, and some of you will find no need to do so, you may call it a *burst*. Notice that the location of the ✳ varies in each cell.

✳	✳	✳
✳	✳	✳
✳	✳	✳

Each ✱ occupies a different combination of top, middle, bottom, left, center, and right of the cell. No two ✱ are in the same location within the cell. You now will observe a sequence of squares and predict the next location of the ✱ in each square. Use T, M, or B to identify the vertical location, and L, C, or R to identify the horizontal location of the ✱. In the following figure, the ✱ is located as:

TL	TC	TR	MR	BR		
✱	✱	✱	✱	✱		

Predict where the next two ✱ would go based on the pattern established. It appears that the ✱ is moving across the top row (TL, TC, TR), down the right column (TR, MR, BR). You may predict that the pattern looks as it appears in the following table. However, you may have identified another pattern altogether!

TL	TC	TR	MR	BR	BC	BL
✱	✱	✱	✱			
				✱	✱	✱

 Visit the Web site www.mentalagility.com for an interactive version of this exercise.

A second type of spatial relationship is rotation of an object. You will consider this in *two dimensions*—that is, on a flat surface, such as this page, and also in three-dimensional space. This is very difficult, and you may find yourself wanting to stop before you arrive at a solution. The advice we can offer that will help you to grow new brain cells is: Keep going! Press on! There *is* an answer, and *you* can find it!

2D Spatial Relationships

Look at the floor plan in Figure 7-5. Which of the other floor plans is a rotation of it?

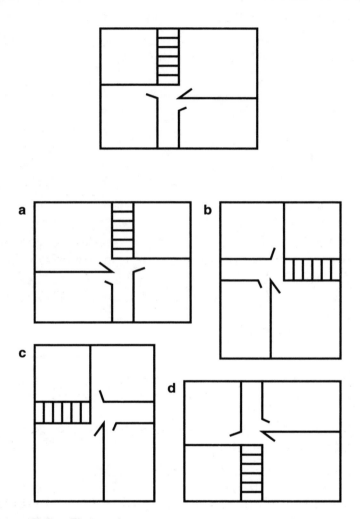

Figure 7-5 Floor plans

The answer is letter **b.** To convince yourself, trace the original plan (you might use the tissue paper that came in a gift box), place it over each of the other plans, and rotate it until it completely matches one of them. To match plan **a, c,** or **d,** flip your tracing paper over and rotate it until it matches plan **a, c,** and **d.** They are the rotations of the mirror image of the original plan.

3D Spatial Relationships

Now consider one of a pair of dice, a die. Use Figure 7-6. Which of the four dice matches the die on the left when rotated?

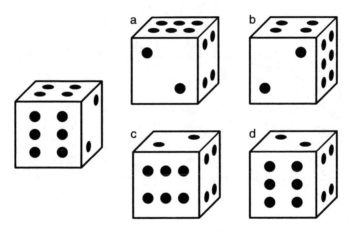

Figure 7-6   Match dice

The answer is letter **a.** It may help to visualize this process:

1. The die on the left was first rolled so that the 6 pips (dots) were on the top.
2. Then it was turned 90 degrees to the left.

It also may help to find a pair of dice and try to set them up to match the picture. As a kinesthetic learner, you will want to turn them in your hands to help verify this result.

Did you notice that all dice are alike in the placement of the pips? That's a standardization you may not have been aware of! Now notice that the dice in options **b, c,** and **d** in the exercise are not even regulation dice. How can you tell? Hint: Try to arrange a die to resemble the dice in b, c, and d.

Another nifty fact about dice is that the opposite sides always add up to seven. That means that the 1 is opposite the 6, the 2 is opposite the 5, and the 3 is opposite the 4. Using this extra fact, along with strategies you learned in the earlier example, find the die on the right that is a copy of the die on the left in Figure 7-7.

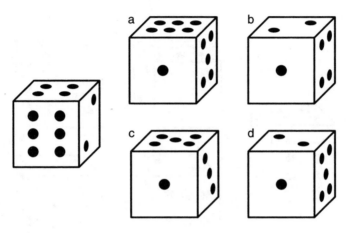

Figure 7-7

Did you select **c?** Visualize the rotation of the die on the left to match the die lettered **c.** First turn the die 180 degrees clockwise until you can see the 1 on the front. Then roll it over on its side, so that the 5 is on top. Now the die matches view **c.** This will take some practice. Use the die if that helps.

You also could solve this puzzle by eliminating incorrect dice. You can eliminate both dice a and d, because they have adjacent (not opposite) faces that add up to seven pips. Additionally, die b has an incorrect face. The two pips on the top face are in the wrong corners. Check this with a regulation die if you like.

Interestingly enough, men generally perform better at this type of activity than women, so women will require a bit more practice to be just as agile with spatial relationships.

 Visit the Web site www.mentalagility.com for an interactive version of this exercise.

Here are some practice exercises for you. Choose the letter of the die that is a rotation of the die on the left.

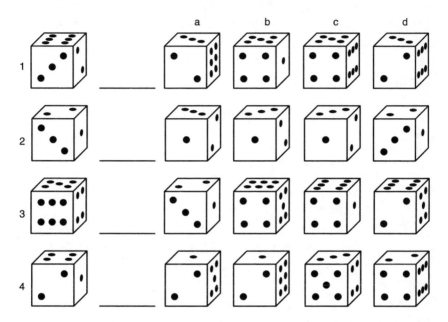

You'll find the answers at the end of this chapter.

Spatial Relationships Exercises

To increase spatial abilities, try to draw a floor plan of your home. After that, sketch a map of your neighborhood. Plan a party where the main activity is a scavenger hunt where you design the field of play. Assemble a model of a vehicle or building that you have admired. In fact, design an activity yourself that will suit your interests. The key components are that you will have to think in three dimensions and create a physical object from parts. The result will be a combination of visual and kinesthetic learning.

ANAGRAMS AND ANAGRAMPS

This is a language exercise. Recall that the visual learning style makes good use of the printed word. Playing word games, in general, will help your language-processing skills and develop your visual learning style.

An *anagram* is a word created from another word by re-arranging all of the letters in the first word. For example, *tar* is an anagram of *rat*. *Art* is also an anagram of *rat* and *tar*. *Danger* is an anagram of *gander*. Try to identify anagrams in the following list.

Identify Anagrams

Are these words anagrams?	Yes	No
1. star rats arts	_____	_____
2. peace piece	_____	_____
3. stare rates tears	_____	_____
4. tub but Btu	_____	_____
5. Easter teaser	_____	_____
6. last first	_____	_____

In this table, lines 1, 3, 4, and 5 contain anagrams. Line 2 contains *homonyms,* words that sound alike. Line 6 contains opposites.

Now that you know what anagrams are, you can try to make some of your own.

What is an anagram of the word *pit?* _____

What is an anagram of the word *bear?* _____

Possible answers include *tip* and *bare*. Did you think of *tip* and *bare?* If so, good for you! Go on to the section named *Play AnaGramps.* If not, let's do some more.

Bonus Exercise

Notice that *bare* is also a homonym for *bear*. Try to find more anagrams that also sound like the original word. This extra exercise will help you work on your *auditory* skills as well.

Let's choose the word *ear*. If you rearrange the letters, you can make new words. Some words you can make are *era* and *are*. You also could rearrange the letters to spell *rea* or *Rae* or *aer*. But these are not words in English. Sometimes *Rae* can be a woman's name, and *aer* means *air* in Irish.

Rearrange these letters to make anagrams:

What is an anagram of the word *spot?* _____

What is an anagram of the word *garden?* _____

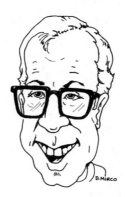

Two of the ones we found for *spot* were *tops* and *pots*. Did you find a third? For *garden,* we can use the anagrams from earlier: *danger* and *gander.*

Play AnaGramps

Now you're ready to play the game. This game is a completion task. Each blank in each sentence can be filled with anagrams.

Sample: I _saw_ a star in the sky as I _was_ walking last night.

AnaGramps

Complete each sentence with an anagram of the word in italics (remember that the sentence must make sense). Try more than once to fill these blanks before checking the answers at the end of this chapter. Each search will strengthen your mind.

1. Pirates used to *rove* _____ the bounding sea.
2. My friend *Thelma* retired to a cottage in a tiny _____ by the sea.
3. The King, *Elvis,* _____. I saw him wearing _____.

Now fill in the blanks with two anagrams.

4. The _____ river is so long and straight that it looks like a _____ on the map.
5. She traveled _____ and far to _____ a living.

6. When he exclaimed "_____!" he didn't _____ to startle you.

7. It is hard to _____ to a _____ movie. That's why they used title frames.

8. Eve was duped by the _____ to _____ Adam with the forbidden fruit.

9. _____ Gonzalez could really _____ during his siesta.

10. The mother bird finally _____ her chicks out of the _____.

11. I pricked my finger on the thorn of a _____ and, boy, is it ever _____!

12. You will need a military _____ if you march through that _____.

13. I _____ the children to stay close and not to _____ off.

14. At _____ I turn on the lights so I won't miss a _____.

15. Read this _____ for me. I want to be sure it has the right _____.

Now that you have the hang of it, try to make up some anagram examples to share with friends. Teach another person how to play AnaGramps, and then trade puzzles.

You can find an anagram by listing all the possible arrangements for a word and then examining each one to determine whether it is a word. For example, *crate* can be re-arranged to form 120 possible words. Here are a few

acert	acetr	acrte	acret	acter	actre
aecrt	aectr	aertc	aerct	aetcr	aetrc
caert	caetr	**carte**	**caret**	**cater**	catre
ceart	ceatr	certa	cerat	cetar	cetra
arect	aretc	arcte	arcet	artec	...

We made 29 arrangements and found only three words! This plan of attack can be exhausting and not much fun. The

CROSSWORD PUZZLE: A Learning style Puzzle

ACROSS

1 Choose from a list
4 Forever youthful
11 Smear test
14 Porcine card game for children
17 Michael Jordan's nickname
18 Chloride (I AM TRUE anagram)
19 Many "I's"
21 Run
22 Auditory learner's "to"
23 Ancient Roman magistrate (A REPORT anagram)
24 Alone
25 Article
26 Scrooge's lament
28 Toss out

30 Swiss mountains
32 Tip over
33 Not far
34 Shortens skirt
37 Pares
40 Flat thin narrow strip
42 A gourd rattle
44 Keep
47 Writing fluid
49 Neurons and glial cells
52 Set up
53 Hydrogen compounds
55 Concious mental state
57 Finish
58 Poly ending (STEER anagram)
60 "A drink with jam and bread..."
61 Money first

64 Visual organ
65 Belonging to me
66 Payable
67 Narcissistic
69 Lack of presence
72 In harmony with
76 Concluding remarks
78 Soiled
79 Peanut candy
80 One billion years
81 Groove
82 Gave temporarily
83 Haute couture
86 Metal or bamboo rods
89 Seed house
92 Astray
94 Yours and mine
95 Tiny disagreement
96 Lives in 30 across

98 Driving aid
99 Concerning the brain
102 Small twitch
103 Title
104 Follows
106 Fence portal
109 Central idea
112 Belts
114 Sandwich fish
116 Noted

119 Grab
120 Blend
121 Wrongly accused
123 For sooth
126 E in HOMES
128 in Hierarchy between
Baron and Knight
131 Tall flightless bird
132 Conflicts
133 Father

134 Nimbleness
135 Contents of 89
across
136 Possess
137 Kinesthetic
acquisition
138 Handworker?
139 Arid

DOWN

1 Promise
2 Holy
3 Tread heavily
4 Holds fluid for injections
(UP A ELM anagram)
5 Auditory output of a
brook
6 Equal Rights
Amendment (abbrev.)
7 Prevaricate
8 Consumed
9 Cookers
10 Sequential
11 Annoyer
12 Before now
13 White bears
14 Tap gently
15 Solid water
16 Bauble
20 Serious
21 Choir step
27 Two footed
29 Crustacean
31 Passage
35 Stirred, not shaken
36 Body of knowledge
38 Citrus

39 Clip
41 Arbor native
43 Consented
44 Took a seat
45 Top card in the deck
46 By way of
48 Last in hierarchy of 128
across
50 Selected at random
51 Product of 55 across
54 Spirit
56 Princess of Wales
59 Refine metals
62 Fishing gear
63 Plunges
66 Passageways
68 Corners
70 Prickly pod
71 Wet snow
72 Evaporate (A TABLE
anagram)
73 Brain condition resulting from alcohol abuse
74 Smallest
75 Devil
77 Not apt
84 Not in

85 Pull
87 Pause
88 Engrave
89 Fruit desert
90 Poem
91 Performed
93 Spread around
97 Dropsy
100 Visual activity
101 Tardy
105 Persuades
107 Knotted hat
108 Promise
110 Worn out
111 Died for a cause
113 Shoot
115 Mountaintop nest
117 Correct
118 Pause
120 Encounter
122 Obligation
123 Another of 22 across
124 Uncooked
126 Vase
127 Anger
129 Mature, wise, arrived
130 Naught

key is to work on developing a strategy that reduces the work and increases the fun. Notice that the bulk of these "words" do not form English words. You can improve your search by developing strategies using what you know about English words. For example, many words start with *tr*, but none with *rt* Find a word starting with *tr*.

This is the type of activity your brain thrives on. When you design your own strategies for playing a game, you exercise your brain in a way it has never been exercised before. Think a while and see whether you can find another strategy for improving your ability to identify an anagram of a word. By the way, *trace* is an anagram of *crate*. Did you find others?

Anagrams can be extended to complete phrases. By rearranging the letters of *Albert Einstein,* Stephen Choi created the anagram *Ten elite brains.* Using a software program named Anagram Genius, Wendy A. Keen found *nice ration size* to be an anagram of *a senior citizen.* Type in *The best things in life are free,* and the program produces the anagram *Nail-biting refreshes the feet*! We found these anagrams at http://www.anagramgenius.com. You can visit the Web site and get a list of anagrams for your name! You also might enjoy the Anagram Hall of Fame at the Web location http://www.wordsmith.org/anagram/hof.html. Samples there include *dormitory* and *dirty room,* as well as *senior moment* and *I'm not Emerson.*

We would like to hear about your strategies for finding anagrams. Go to this book's Web site at http://www. mentalagility.com. Access the Anagrams and Anagramps menu item and send us your ideas. We'll post new strategies for other readers to read and use. You also will find an option on the Web page for letting us know about AnaGramps you have created. We'll post the first ones we receive from each reader.

This is an interesting note for math lovers on the possible number of arrangements of a set of letters in a word. The number of arrangements of letters in a word of all different letters is calculated by a formula known as a *factorial.* Suppose that there are five letters in a word. Imagine five blanks: _ _ _ _ _ . Where might you place the first letter? You have five choices. Then there are only four places left for the second letter, three for the third letter, two for the fourth letter, and then only one place remains for the last letter. Multiply $5 \times 4 \times 3 \times 2 \times 1$. The result is 120. Mathematicians devised shorthand for writing out this problem: 5!. The exclamation point is read as "factorial." 5! is read as "5 factorial." So $4! = 4 \times 3 \times 2 \times 1$. And 7! is $7 \times 6 \times 5 \times 4 \times 3 \times 2 \times 1$. If no letters are repeated, the number of possible rearrangements for a word with n letters is $n!$

WORD FIT! A FILL-IN PUZZLE

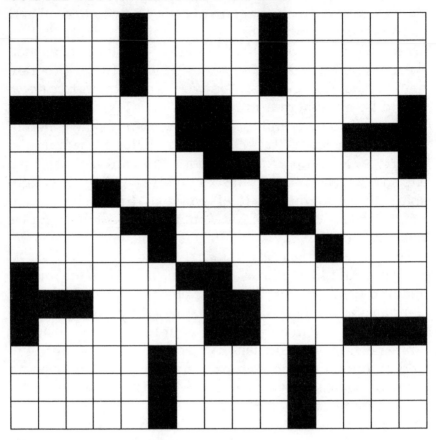

In this puzzle you have all of the words. To solve the puzzle, put all the words in their proper location. (Hint: Since there are only two 8-letter words, try to place them first.)

3 LETTERS

ADO
ALL
ALP
BAY
EBB
EGO
EVE
FAT
GAP
GIN
ITS
LIE
LOB
MAN
MOB
PEN
SEE
SUE
TED
TOE

4 LETTERS

ABET
AIRY
ASIA
AXON
CLIP
EASY
EBBS
ENDS
ETCH
EYED
FLAP
GLUE
LOBE
NAVE
NEAT
NILE
OBOE
OLEO
OMEN
PEAS
RODE
SINS
SLAB
TOOT

5 LETTERS

ALIGN
AMASS
ARISE
CLING
DIALS
ENACT
FILAR
PEEPS
PIXIE
PRIME
PRONE
SLANT
STOLE
THESE
TYPED
WIPED

6 LETTERS

ACCEPT
ENCORE
IRENIC
MATTER
PAEANS
SANDAL
SOIREE
TISANE
WISEST
YEOMEN

7 LETTERS

APPEARS
COSINES
FRONTAL
IRANIAN
SNEERED
TOOTERS

8 LETTERS

MIRABILE
SLIPCASE

WORD UP!

Find the message hidden in these letters. Rearrange the letters below and place them in the grid to make a sentence. We'll give you a hint! The letters are already in the correct columns.

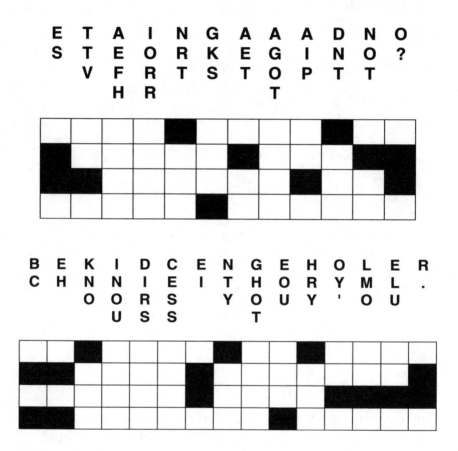

MIND MATCHES

Many words are used in technical ways that are related to the original etymology of a word. The etymology of a word is similar to its pedigree. It describes the origin of the word, in what languages it was used, and how its meaning has changed over the years.

The object of this game is to match each word with its origin. Some matches are more obvious than others. This game develops your verbal comprehension, which is one of the skills tested on an IQ test. For this game, we encourage you to use a dictionary. You will find many wonderful new words in your dictionary as you try to solve this puzzle. Answers are at the end of this chapter.

Match each brain-related use of the following terms with their word origins.

1. ___ homunculus
2. ___ circadian
3. ___ hippocampus

4. ___ rehearsal
5. ___ neurons
6. ___ hemisphere
7. ___ auditory
8. ___ temporal
9. ___ lobes
10. ___ thalamus
11. ___ reticular system
12. ___ limbic system
13. ___ glial
14. ___ kinesthetic
15. ___ synapse
16. ___ cortex

a. glue-like
b. juncture
c. a half of the celestial sphere of stars and planets
d. rounded body parts
e. bark
f. nerves
g. relating to time
h. a little human
i. opposite of anesthetic
j. chamber
k. to cultivate again
l. related to hearing
m. about a day
n. border area of the cortex
o. sea horse
p. similar to a pouch or a woman's drawstring bag

THE CALENDAR

The calendar is a tool we use every day, and it is so common you probably don't ever think much about its origins. It helps to think about it as a human creation. This set of exercises helps to develop your verbal fluency. An almanac is a handy tool for this job.

"Remember that time is money." — *Benjamin Franklin*

The Vocabulary of the Calendar

Look in an almanac to find out the *etymology*, or the origins of the words, for the following terms: calendar, day, week, month, year, Sunday, Monday, Tuesday, Wednesday, Thursday, Friday, Saturday, January, February, March, April, May, June, July, August, September, October, November, December.

Calendar Reform

Currently we follow the Gregorian calendar. Use an almanac to find out how our current calendar was developed. If you are interested in genealogy, you know about the calendar reform of 1582 finally adopted by the British in 1752. If not, find out about calendar reform. Try to determine why there are 12 months of uneven numbers of days. It seems like an arbitrary decision for breaking up the 365 days.

Calendars of Other Cultures

Investigate the Chinese calendar. How is it like the Gregorian calendar? How is it different? Investigate other calendars for other groups.

How Many Calendars Do You Ever Need?

Have you noticed that many years have the same arrangements of dates? For example, the calendar for the year 2000 is the same one we used in 1972. How many different calendars do you need to keep around so that you always have a correct version? When is the next time you will be able to use the 1999 calendar again? Answers for this question are at the end of this chapter.

Day of the Week Calculation

Ever wonder on what day of the week you were born? Find out the day of the week for any date after 1753. Use the following calculation. We will demonstrate with February 6, 1897. The last column is provided for you to work this calculation on a date of your choosing.

Steps	Step #	Sample Values	Your Values
Write the day of the month.	1	6	
Write the month.	2	2	
Write the year.	3	1897	
If the month is January or February, add 1 to the number in step 1.	4	7	
If the month is January or February, subtract 1 from the number in step 3.	5	1896	
Write the first two digits of the number in step 5.	6	18	
Divide the number in step 6 by 4. (Toss the remainder.)	7	4	
Multiply the number in step 3 by 5.	8	9485	
Divide the number in step 8 by 4. (Toss the remainder.)	9	2371	
Add 1 to the number in step 5.	10	1897	
Multiply the number in step 10 by 13.	11	24661	
Divide the number in step 11 by 5. (Toss the remainder.)	12	4932	
Add the numbers in steps 9 and 12.	13	7303	
Subtract the number in step 7 from the number in step 13.	14	7299	
Add the number in step 6 to the number in step 14.	15	7317	
Add the number in step 1 to the number in step 15.	16	7323	
Subtract 1 from the number in step 16.	17	7322	
Divide the number in step 17 by 7. *Keep* only the remainder.	18	0	

The number in step 18 tells you on which day of the week 2/6/1987 fell. Use this table to determine the name of the day of the week:

Remainder	Decimal part of answer (if you used a calculator)	Day of the Week
1	0.14285714...	Sunday
2	0.28571428...	Monday
3	0.42857142...	Tuesday
4	0.57142857...	Wednesday
5	0.71428571...	Thursday
6	0.85714285...	Friday
0	0	Saturday

So, February 6, 1897 was on a Saturday. Try this calculation with a date of your choice.

Number of Days in Each Month

You may recall the jingle for remembering the number of days in each month. "Thirty days hath September, April, June, and November. All the rest have 31, except February." This is an example of a mnemonic device. This works very well for an auditory learner. However, a kinesthetic or visual learner may experience difficulty remembering the order of the months in that device. A visual learner may remember the number of days in a month by remembering what a calendar looks like. For a kinesthetic learner, there is another way to remember the number of days in a month. It uses your hands as a tool. Make a pair of fists, as shown in Figure 7-8.

Notice that your knuckles form peaks and valleys. Start at the left hand, first knuckle, and recite the months of the year, in order, using peaks and valleys. When you run out of knuckles on your left hand, go to your right hand for August on the first knuckle. Continue until you reach December. Notice that all of the months you named by a knuckle have 31 days. Those you named by a valley do not. All of those months, except February, have 30 days. Most people remember about February.

As an exercise, explain this calendar mechanism to someone. Tell him it is a great mnemonic device—a handy digital device, solar powered, and pocket-sized.

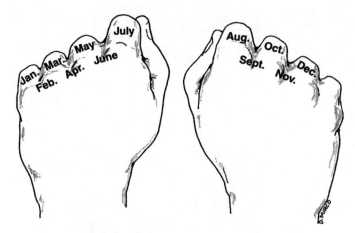

Figure 7-8 Knuckle calendar

A Very Spatial Puzzle

Copy these patterns to a piece of cardstock or a 3"× 5" card. Cut out the pieces and rearrange the smaller pieces to make the big square. Hint: Flip the puzzle pieces over if it helps.

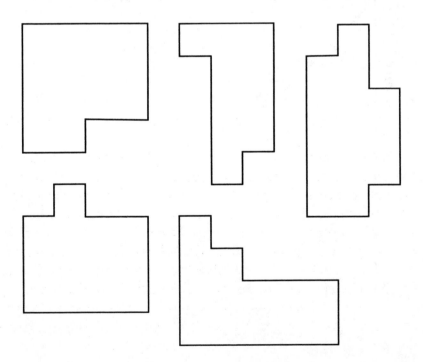

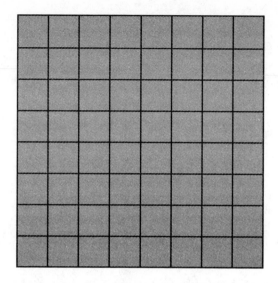

THE HOUSE THAT JACK BUILT

For this exercise, you'll use Figure 7-9. An ancient Chinese puzzle called *tangrams* will improve your kinesthetic learning

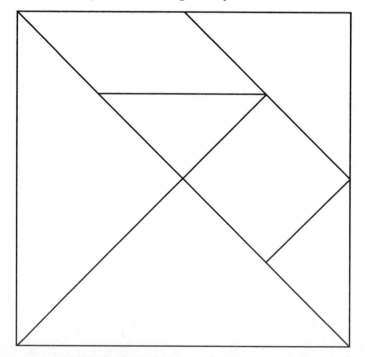

Figure 7-9 Chinese tans

skills. The puzzle pieces, or *tans,* all are cut from a square. Then the tans are arranged in shapes by puzzle masters. A silhouette is drawn and given to a puzzler to solve. The puzzler rearranges the seven tans to match the arrangements.

You can learn ancient puzzle techniques. Using a blank piece of paper, trace Figure 7-9. Cut out all seven tans. Spend some time noticing the seven pieces. Some are alike, some are very different. For your first puzzle, put the seven tans back into a square. Don't peek at the diagram on this page!

After you master the square puzzle, you can move on to a set of puzzles. This is a puzzle made to match the characters in a famous old nursery rhyme, *The House That Jack Built.*

This is the House that Jack built.

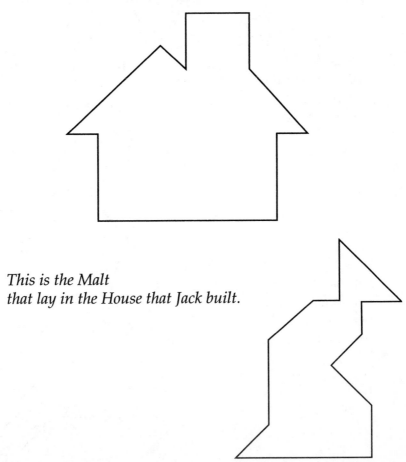

This is the Malt
that lay in the House that Jack built.

This is the Rat
that ate the Malt
that lay in the House that Jack built.

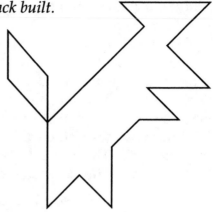

This is the Cat
that killed the Rat
that ate the Malt
that lay in the House that Jack built.

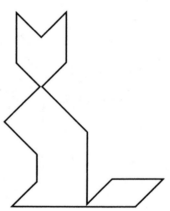

This is the Dog
that worried the Cat
that killed the Rat
that ate the Malt
that lay in the House that Jack built.

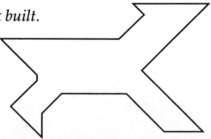

This is the Cow with the Crumpled Horn
that tossed the Dog
that worried the Cat
that killed the Rat
that ate the Malt
that lay in the House that Jack built.

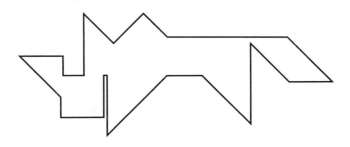

This is the Maiden all forlorn
that milked the cow with the crumpled horn
that tossed the Dog
that worried the Cat
that killed the Rat
that ate the Malt
that lay in the House that Jack built.

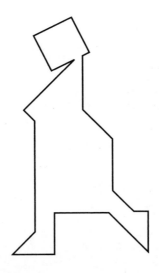

This is the Man all tattered and torn
that kissed the Maiden all forlorn
that milked the cow with the crumpled horn
that tossed the Dog
that worried the Cat
that killed the Rat
that ate the Malt
that lay in the House that Jack built.

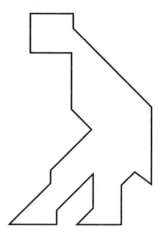

This is the Priest all shaven and shorn
that married the Man all tattered and torn
that kissed the Maiden all forlorn
that milked the cow with the crumpled horn
that tossed the Dog
that worried the Cat
that killed the Rat
that ate the Malt
that lay in the House that Jack built.

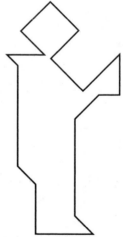

This is the Cock that crowed in the morn
that waked the Priest all shaven and shorn
that married the Man all tattered and torn
that kissed the Maiden all forlorn
that milked the cow with the crumpled horn
that tossed the Dog
that worried the Cat
that killed the Rat
that ate the Malt
that lay in the House that Jack built.

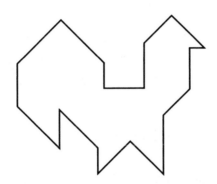

BOXER REBELLION

 Making common objects can help you develop spatial-relationship skills. Suppose that you want to make a box. The following patterns are ways you can arrange five sides of a box on a piece of cardboard. Some of them can be folded up to make a box without a lid. Some cannot. Try to determine which can and which cannot. You'll find answers at the end of this chapter.

 Use Figure 7-10. If your dominant style is visual or auditory, copy these patterns to grid paper and then cut them out. Try to fold them up to make a box. This exercise will help develop your kinesthetic skills.

 If kinesthetic is your dominant style, try to visualize which patterns can be folded to make the box without touching the patterns. You may make sketches on a notepad, if you like, but no touching!

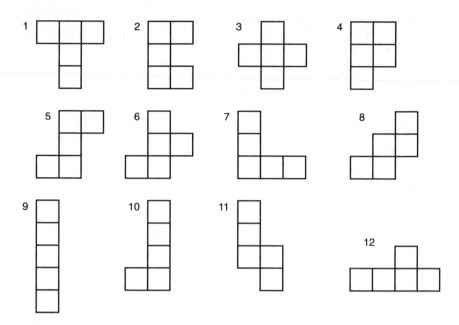

Figure 7-10 Boxer Rebellion I

A box may not be very helpful without a lid, so Figure 7-11 contains patterns of six squares that may or may not be helpful in making a box with its lid. Determine which can and which cannot be folded into a box with a lid. Answers are at the end of this chapter.

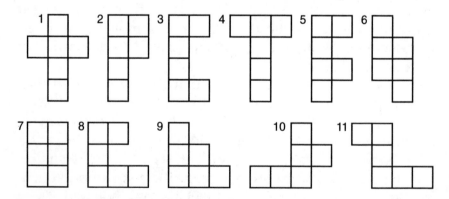

Figure 7-11 Boxer Rebellion 2

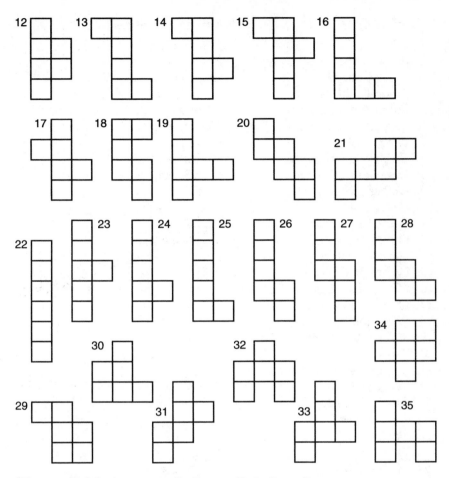

Figure 7-11 (continued) Boxer Rebellion 2

TOOL SCHOOLS

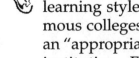 This is a set of puns to help you improve your auditory learning style. Listen to the sounds of the names of the famous colleges and universities as you match them up with an "appropriate" major for a degree fancifully offered by the institution. For example, Albright College suggests the homonym "all bright." Look for a degree having to do with brightness. You would choose Lighting Engineer.

Tool Schools

1. Albright College
2. Barry University
3. Bates College
4. Bloomfield College
5. Butler University
6. Campbell University
7. Colby College
8. Colgate University
9. Dartmouth College
10. DePauw University
11. Drew University
12. Drexel University
13. Duke University
14. Lincoln College
15. Lycoming College
16. Morehouse College
17. Oxford University
18. Princeton University
19. Stetson University
20. Tulane University
21. University of Charleston
22. Webber State College
23. Yale University

Degree Offered

____ Agriculture
____ Art
____ Automotive Engineering
____ Boxing
____ Construction
____ Cotton Shirt Manufacturing
____ Dance
____ DeVeterinarian
____ Domestications
____ Fishing
____ Furniture Design
____ Grilling
____ Haberdashery
____ Highway Design
____ Horticulture
____ Hotel Management
____ Lighting Engineer
____ Locksmith
____ Prevarication
____ Regal Studies
____ Soupmaking
____ Dentistry
____ Undertaker

SO I SAYS . . .

 This exercise was invented by Keith Harmeyer and his former student, Lee Steer, as they conversed while Lee was in college. At the end of each letter, Keith would add a new So I Says, and in return, Lee would add one to her letters. You can use this game to build your auditory learning skills.

In each of the following lines, you can respond by selecting a name that sounds like a word that is described by the first part of the sentence. For example: If I were to say to you, "So I says to the guy changing his tire, I says, Jack!" You would realize that a jack is used to change a tire and it is the name of a person. The coincidence of sounds introduces humor, we hope. Your job is to notice how many words sound like common names. The answers are at the end of this chapter.

1. So I says to the girl blessing the food, I says . . .

_____

2. So I says to the man headed to physical education, I says . . . _____

3. So I says to the kid playing with his trains, I says . . .

_____

4. So I says to the girl watching the sunrise, I says . . .

_____

5. So I says to the girl taking me to court, I says . . .

_____

6. So I says to the guy using the PA system, I says . . .

_____

7. So I says to the woman making hamburgers, I says . . .

_____

8. So I says to the fellow saying his prayers, I says . . .

_____

9. So I says to the boy doing subtraction problems, I says . . . _____

10. So I says to the fellow floating gently on the waves, I says . . . _____

11. So I says to the guy getting dressed, I says . . .

_____

12. So I says to the lady drinking Harvey's Bristol Cream, I says . . . _____

13. So I says to the fellow who thinks carnival games are fair, I says . . .

_____

14. So I says to the man seasoning the sauce, I says . . .

_____

15. So I says to da sister of da nephew, I says . . .

_____

16. So I says to the guy who just hit the lottery, I says . . .

_____

17. So I says to the man learning to tame lions, I says . . .

    _____

18. So I says to the two guys with the drums, I says . . .

    _____

19. So I says to the two girls working in the fabric store, I says . . . _____

20. So I says to the guy looking a little pale, I says . . .

    _____

 Now that you have completed this exercise, you may have created a few "So I says" of your own. Let us know by sending e-mail to puzzles@mentalagility.com. You can also visit the web site www.mentalagility.com and add one more to the list on the site.

NINE-DOT PROBLEM

 There is a classic problem that works on your visual learning style as well as your creativity and spatial-relationship skills. It is called the Nine Dot problem because it is concerned with the following array of dots:

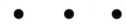

The task is to connect the dots with four straight lines without taking the pencil off the page. No line should double back over another line. Each dot must be on at least one line. After you try this, check the answer at the end of this chapter.

GLUTTON

This game improves your ability to concentrate. You will need a pair of dice and an opponent. The object of the game is to roll the dice as many times as you like on your turn, adding up the pips on the dice with the goal of eventually reaching 100. However, if you roll a 1 on either die, your score stays the same. If you roll *snake eyes* (a 2), your turn is over and your score reverts to 0. Otherwise, add the total of the pips to your score. End your turn when you decide to or if you roll snake eyes. Then the other person begins to roll the dice. The first person to reach 100 wins.

Try to predict when you might roll snake eyes. Determine how likely it is to roll them. Develop a strategy for winning this game. If you are lucky, you can get to 100 on one turn without rolling snake eyes. How much luck do you think there is in this game? Can you compensate with a clever strategy? How lucky do you feel today?

At the beginning, you may want to use a paper and pencil to keep the totals. As you increase your concentration powers, you will want to keep the totals in your head, for both players.

FIGURE AND GROUND

Whenever a figure is drawn in a frame, the space becomes divided into two sections: the figure (or foreground) and the ground (or background). For some highly visual people with great spatial-relationship skills, the figure and ground readily change places. Consider the drawing in Figure 7-12.

Let's say this figure shows steps in your home. Are you looking at them from above or from below? It depends on what part of the picture your mind assigns to the background and what part it assigns to the foreground. When the foreground is in the lower left corner, it appears that the steps are below you. However, if you can make your brain decide that the foreground is in the upper right, it appears that the steps are above you, as if you were standing on a basement step looking up.

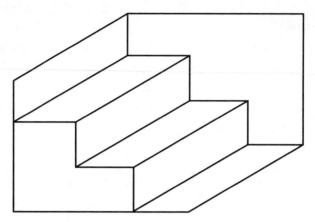

Figure 7-12 Example of Figure and Ground

This same phenomenon applies to these stylized silhouettes of people in Figure 7-13. Here, no frame contains the space, and the black comes to the foreground. Stare at the pictures in Figure 7-13 for a while.

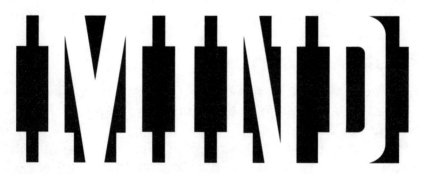

Figure 7-13 Example of Figure and Ground

It may take some time to push the black blobs into the background to see the figure in the foreground. What appears is a familiar word in white letters on a black background.

NIM GOLF

 To improve your kinesthetic learning style, use golf tees to play this game. Some people used matchsticks when they were a staple of every kitchen. NIM is an ancient game of skill. To begin, place four tees in a pile, then place two in another pile, and place one in a pile of its own.

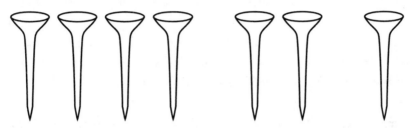

Figure 7-14 Ancient game of NIM using golf tees

Play with another person. The object of this game is to take the last tee. On each turn, you may take one, two, or three tees from any one pile. Try to make the other player take the last tee. Develop a strategy to increase the number of wins.

MATH MAGIC

Here's a quick exercise to accomplish. Improve your problem-solving skills by trying to determine how this trick works.

Write down a three-digit number. _____

Multiply it by 11. _____

Multiply it by 13. _____

Multiply it by 7. _____

Describe the answer. How does that work?

OK, here's another trick: Write down number that represents the month of your birthday. (2, for February, 3 for March, etc.) _____

Multiply it by 5. _____

Add 8. _____

Multiply by 4. _____

Add 3. _____
Multiply by 5. _____
Add the day (date) of the month of your birthday. _____
Subtract 175. _____

What do you see? The first one or two digits of your answer should be your birth month, and the last two should be your birth day. How does this work? At first, use a calculator to do this trick. Improve your concentration skills by practicing it mentally.

You can try this with your friends. This is a clever way to find out a birthday that you think you should know without asking the other person what it is!

MENTAL AGILITY POSTTEST

Now that you have practiced and learned new problem-solving skills, you are ready to take the postassessment. Again, set a timer for 10 minutes. Look for the next item in each pattern.

When the time is up, check your answers. Count the number you answered correctly, and compare your score with your pretest score.

_____ 1. 1, 4, 7, 10, **?**

_____ 2.

_____ 3.

_____ 4. 1, 0, 2, 0, 3, **?**

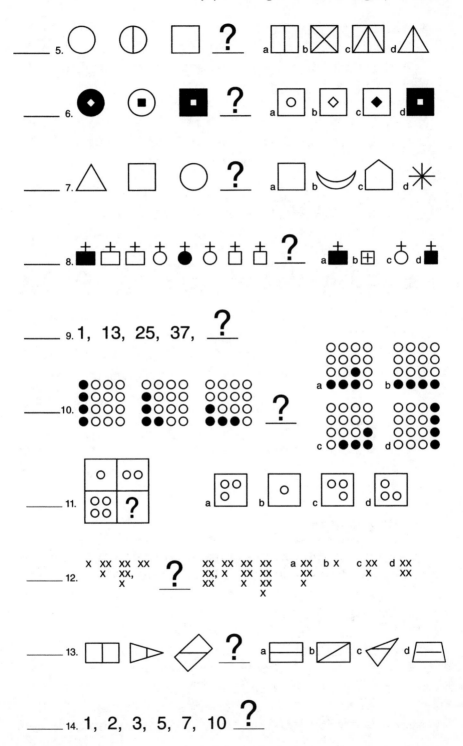

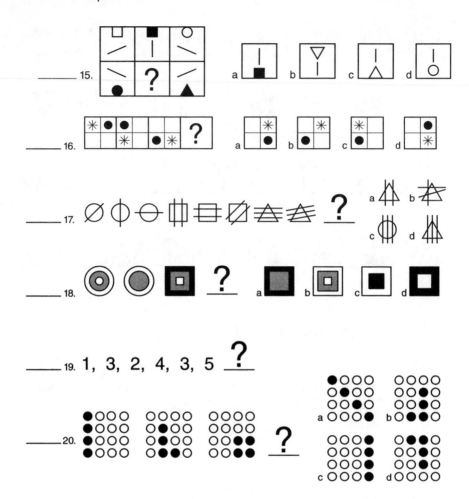

_____ 15.

_____ 16.

_____ 17.

_____ 18.

_____ 19. 1, 3, 2, 4, 3, 5 _?_

_____ 20.

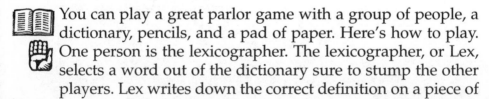

MORE GAMES

Keep using your brain in new and novel ways. Here are a few games you can learn to play with others.

PLAY WORDSMITH

You can play a great parlor game with a group of people, a dictionary, pencils, and a pad of paper. Here's how to play. One person is the lexicographer. The lexicographer, or Lex, selects a word out of the dictionary sure to stump the other players. Lex writes down the correct definition on a piece of paper. Each of the other players creates a fictional definition for the obscure word on a separate piece of paper. Then Lex collects the papers and shuffles the papers. Lex reads each definition. Each player selects the definition he or she thinks is correct. Scoring is based on how well you fool other players and how difficult the word is that Lex selects. Lex gets one point for every player who did not choose the correct definition. All players get one point for every player who chose their definition, and one point if they guess the correct definition. That constitutes one round. Play enough rounds so that each player has a chance to be Lex. There are hilarious moments. Hearing people's definitions for words about which they have no clue can be a hoot. This game is sure to help your auditory skills by practicing your concentration on the reading of the definitions.

Some wonderful words spawn some clever, albeit incorrect, definitions. Here are a few real definitions:

bon'te bok, *n.* a species of purplish-red antelope of South Africa

flot, *n.* scum, floating grease, as in fatty broth

moff, *n.* a light silk fabric woven in the Caucasus

my'ta cism, *n.* abnormally frequent or incorrect use of the letter m

It would be very difficult to believe that these were the correct definitions for these otherwise normal-sounding words! You will find yourself browsing the dictionary looking for the best word to use the next time you play Wordsmith.

MAGIC MENTAL MINUTES

Building mental agility does not have to be an all-consuming event. You can do many things that take just a minute and will work cumulatively to increase your mental abilities:

- Look up a word in a dictionary. While you are reading or watching TV, a word will come up for which you may not know the meaning. Take one minute to look it up in the dictionary.

- Mentally review the names of the people you met at the last social event you attended. Match their names and faces with a fact you found out about them.

- Add the digits on the license plate in front of you at a traffic light. Then multiply the digits. Decide which is greater, the sum or the product.

- Add the digits of the license plate. Then add the digits of that sum. Continue adding until your sum is a single digit. Then divide the license plate number by 9. The remainder, if any, will be the same as that single digit.

- Determine the best poker hand from the numbers on the license plate of a van.

- If there are letters on the license plate, see how many words you can form that have the letters in the same order, in reverse order, in any order. For example, if a license tag has the letters AFD on it, you can find the name **Alfredo**.

- If there are letters on the license plate, create an acrostic for the letters. An *acrostic* is a sentence in which each word begins with a letter in the list. For example, if a license tag has the letters AFD on it, make up a sentence such as **A**rnold **f**eeds **d**ogs.

Caution: Do not perform any of these license-tag activities while your car is moving, unless you are a passenger!

- Look at a scene, say, in a picture or out of doors. Close your eyes and try to recall as many of the objects in the scene as you can for one minute. Try this specifically with a room in your home.

- Look at that same scene and find connections among the items in the scene. How many objects are trees? How many are manmade, and so on.

- Pick up a crossword puzzle from the newspaper and try to fill in just one word.

- At the checkout counter, if you are purchasing just one item, try to predict the amount of the sales tax. To do this, you will have to be in a state where sales tax is assessed, and you will have to know the tax rate. Alternatively, after you give the cashier your money, predict the amount of change you should receive.

- Deal a deck of cards into eight piles. Predict the number of face cards in each stack. Look at one stack to see whether your prediction was correct. Predict how many face cards are in each of the remaining stacks. Continue guessing and looking at the remaining stacks one by one, and refine your prediction each time for the stacks that remain.

- Figure out another route to take from your home to the market. Next time you go to the market, take that route. Alternatively, map out a new route for your next walk. Write down the directions, if you like. (Did you know that this is actually a suggestion made by police officers for your safety?)

- See how may words you can create using the letters in your name in one minute.

- While watching TV, look at a one-minute commercial and determine what the downside or upside is to purchasing the product being advertised.

- While watching TV, decide whether the last action of the hero or heroine is "in character." Predict the outcome of the conversation or action presented.

- Tune in to a quiz show and try to answer a few questions.

- Keep a jigsaw puzzle set up if you have the space. Spend one minute looking for one piece of the puzzle.

- Pull out seven Scrabble™ tiles and try to make the longest word you can in one minute.

- Scan a newspaper for a certain word, say, *the*. Count how many times you can find the word *the* on the front page in one minute. Don't overlook words such as wea**ther**!

- Make one entry in a journal. Reminisce about a childhood event. Build a written history of your life one minute at a time.

- Respell a three-letter word in alphabetical order. For example, the word *get* spelled alphabetically is *egt; tar* respelled is *art.* Notice that some respellings form actual words. After you achieve success with three-letter words, move up to four-letter words.

- Make a mental picture of five of your friends. Rethink the picture so that the youngest is on the left and the oldest is on the right. Then order all of your friends by age. Try this again arranging them from shortest to tallest.

- Draw a rough view of your home. Try to locate the plants, bushes, or trees around the building without looking.

- Name all the credit cards or photos in your wallet or purse. Check later for accuracy.

- If you read the comics section of your newspaper, name five comic strips. Give yourself extra credit for naming the cartoonists.

Caution! This list is not intended for performing in one sitting. You should use it as a resource when you are looking for a one-minute mental task. After practicing with this list, you will be able to invent your own Magic Mental Minutes. Visit the companion Web page for this book, www.mentalagility.com, and let us know what you have invented.

AMAZING MAZES

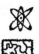

This set of mazes develops visual and kinesthetic abilities, as well as problem-solving skills. Start with the smaller mazes and work up to the more complex. What you learn in earlier mazes, you can apply to the more complex.

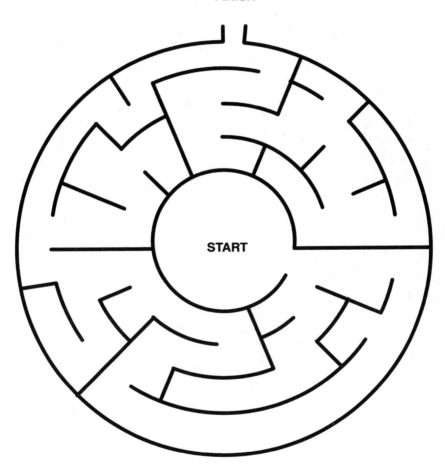

Maze I

FINISH

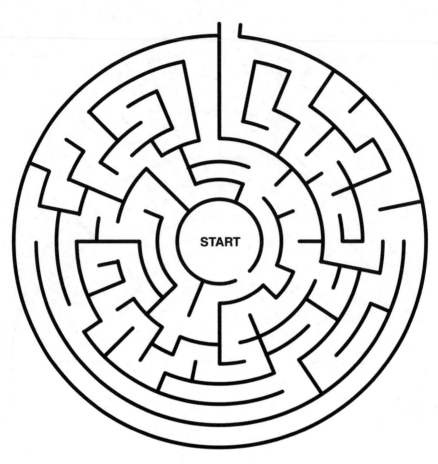

Maze 2

FINISH

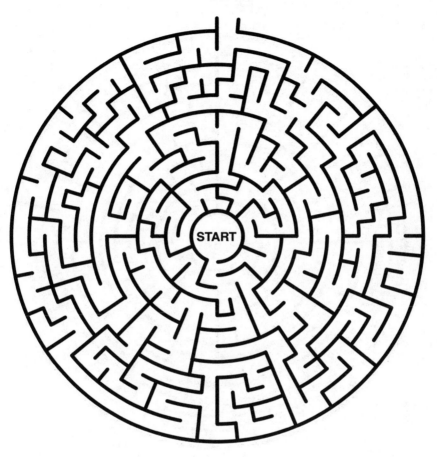

Maze 3

FINISH

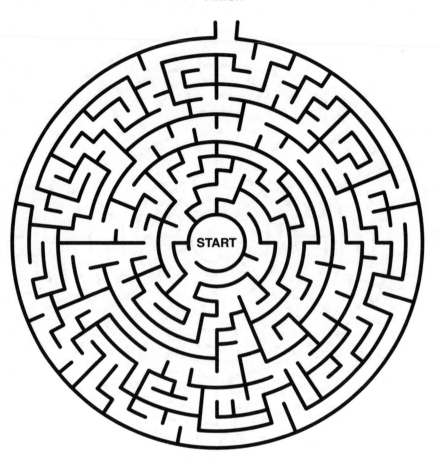

Maze 4

FINISH

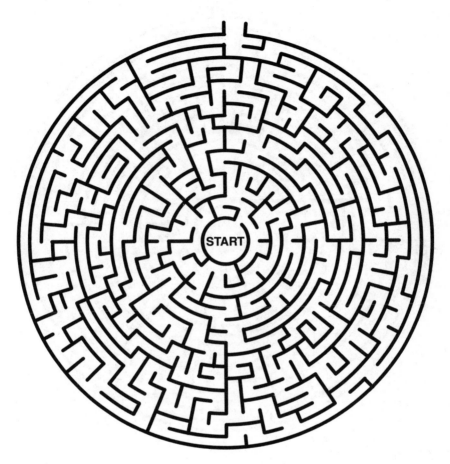

Maze 5

FINISH

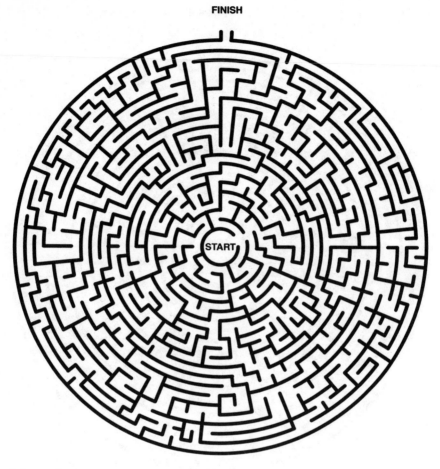

Maze 6

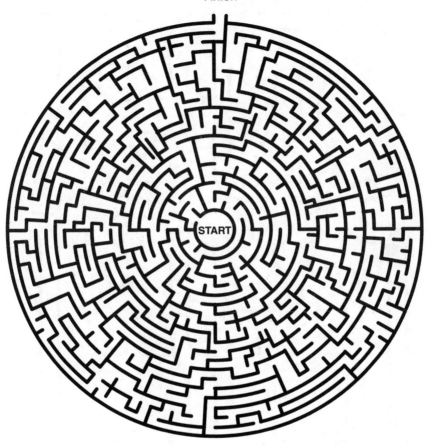

Maze 7

FINISH

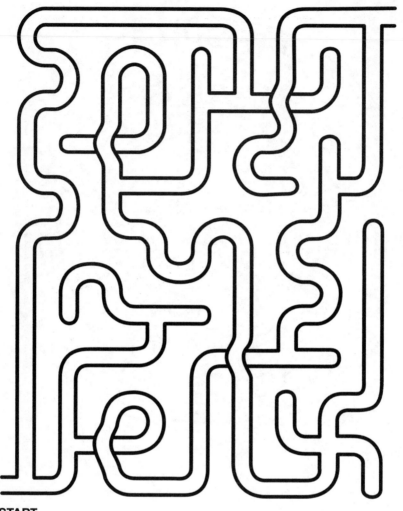

START

Maze 8

FINISH

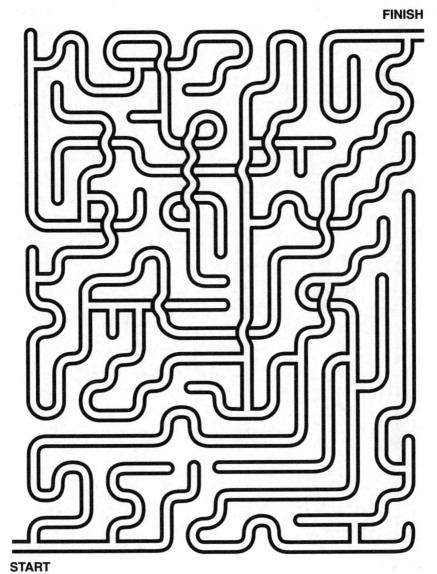

START

Maze 9

FINISH

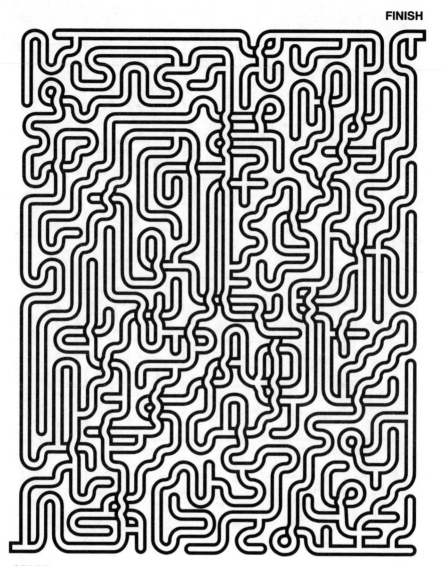

START

Maze 10

CONCLUSION

The only person you can change is yourself. Get out there and grow some brain cells—start today!

ANSWERS

Mental Agility Pretest

 1. J   2. c   3. d   4. 15   5. a   6. c   7. b   8. c   9. 36   10. b
11. a **12.** a **13.** d **14.** 81 **15.** a **16.** b **17.** b **18.** a **19.** 5
20. d

Exercises

Division Quotient

$1/7 = 0.142857142857\ldots$
$2/7 = 0.285714285714\ldots$
$3/7 = 0.428571428571$
$4/7 = 0.571428571428$
$5/7 = 0.714285714285\ldots$
$6/7 = 0.857142857142\ldots$

Sequence of Letters

The sequence A, E, F, H, . . . is the sequence of uppercase letters that can be drawn with only straight lines. So, the next such letter is I.

Inductive Reasoning Exercises

1. 17; Add 4 to each term to find the next term.

2. P; Every third letter of the alphabet.

3. 5; Subtract 1, subtract 2, subtract 3, subtract 4.

4. 16; Even numbers alternate with odd numbers.

5. 5; Divide each term by 5 to find the next term.

6. J; First letter of the months of the year.

7. 125; $1 \times 1 \times 1 = 1$, $2 \times 2 \times 2 = 8$, $3 \times 3 \times 3 = 27$, $4 \times 4 \times 4 = 64$, $5 \times 5 \times 5 = 125$. Or $1^3, 2^3, 3^3, 4^3, 5^3$.

8. 100001; Insert another 0 for each term.

9. O; The letters of the alphabet we use round strokes to draw.

10. Y; A tough one. The letters of the top row of a standard keyboard.

Match Dice

1. a **2.** b **3.** br **4.** d

AnaGramps

1. over **2.** hamlet **3.** Elvis, lives, Levis **4.** Nile, line **5.** near, earn **6.** amen, mean **7.** listen, silent **8.** serpent, present **9.** Señor, snore **10.** sent, nest **11.** rose, sore **12.** escort, sector **13.** warned, wander **14.** night, thing **15.** note, tone

Word Puzzles

Crossword Puzzle

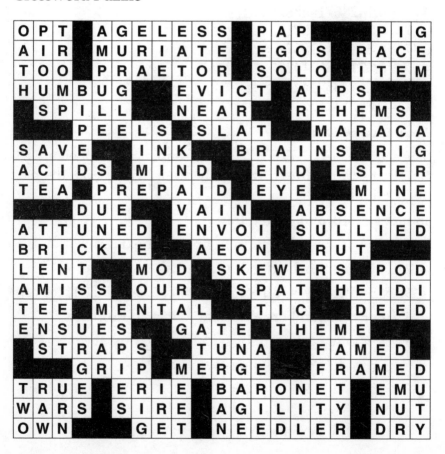

Word Fit! A Fill-In Puzzle

E	A	S	Y		F	L	A	P		A	M	A	S	S
G	L	U	E		R	O	D	E		P	I	X	I	E
O	L	E	O		O	B	O	E		P	R	O	N	E
			M	A	N		P	A	E	A	N	S		
W	I	S	E	S	T		S	L	A	B				
I	R	A	N	I	A	N		P	R	I	M	E		
P	E	N		A	L	I	G	N		S	L	A	N	T
E	N	D	S		L	I	E			E	T	C	H	
D	I	A	L	S		E	N	A	C	T		T	O	E
	C	L	I	N	G		T	O	O	T	E	R	S	
	P	E	A	S		S	O	I	R	E	E			
A	C	C	E	P	T		I	T	S					
F	I	L	A	R		O	M	E	N		A	B	E	T
A	R	I	S	E		L	O	B	E		N	A	V	E
T	Y	P	E	D		E	B	B	S		E	Y	E	D

Word Up!

E	V	E	R		S	T	O	P		T	O
	T	H	I	N	K		A	N	D		
		F	O	R	G	E	T		T	O	
S	T	A	R	T		A	G	A	I	N	?

B	E		N	I	C	E		T	O		Y	O	U	R
		K	I	D	S		T	H	E	Y	'	L	L	
C	H	O	O	S	E		Y	O	U	R				
	N	U	R	S	I	N	G		H	O	M	E	.	

Mind Matches

1. h **2.** m **3.** o **4.** k **5.** f **6.** c **7.** l **8.** g
9. d **10.** j **11.** p **12.** n **13.** a **14.** i **15.** b **16.** e

How Many Calendars Do You Ever Need?

4. There are only 14 different calendars. After a year starts, there are only two options for the rest of the days. Either the year is a leap year and there is an extra day in February, or it is not a leap year. So, we need seven different calendars for a leap year and seven more for a non–leap year. To investigate further, use the words "perpetual calendar" to aid in your search.

The year 1999 started on a Friday. It is the same calendar we used in 1993. The next non–leap year that starts on a Friday is 2010. Save your old 1999 calendar and use it again in 2010. The year 2000 calendar gets a rerun in 2028.

Boxer Rebellion

These figures make boxes without lids: 1, 3, 5, 6, 8, 10, 11, 12. These figures make boxes with lids: 1, 4, 13, 14, 15, 17, 20, 21, 27, 31, 33.

Tool Schools

7, 11, 14, 13, 16, 17, 21, 10, 5, 9, 12, 22, 19, 20, 4, 3, 1, 23, 15, 18, 6, 8, 2

So I Says . . .

1. Grace **2.** Jim (Gym) **3.** Lionel **4.** Dawn **5.** Sue **6.** Mike (microphone) **7.** Patty **8.** Neil (kneel) **9.** Les (less) **10.** Bob **11.** Don **12.** Sherry **13.** Mark **14.** Herb **15.** Denise **16.** Rich **17.** Claude **18.** Tom, Tom **19.** Polly, Esther (polyester) **20.** Juan (wan)

Nine-Dot Problem

The key to this problem is to visualize the space outside the nine dots and use it. This problem is the origin of the now popular phrase *thinking outside the box.*

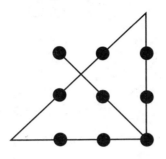

Mental Agility Posttest

1. 13   **2.** b   **3.** c   **4.** 0   **5.** a   **6.** b   **7.** a   **8.** d   **9.** 49   **10.** b
11. c   **12.** d   **13.** c   **14.** 13   **15.** c   **16.** a   **17.** d   **18.** a
19. 4   **20.** c

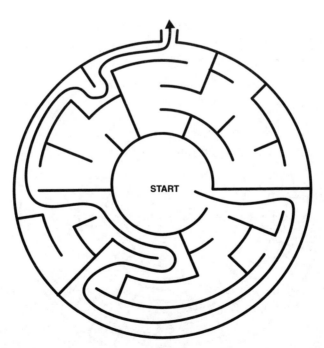

Maze I

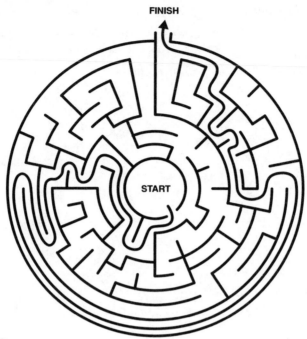

Maze 2

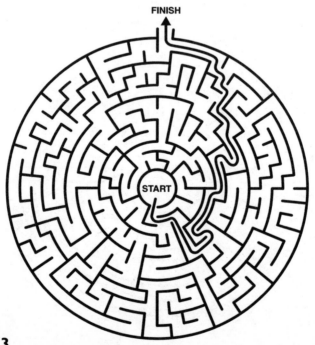

Maze 3

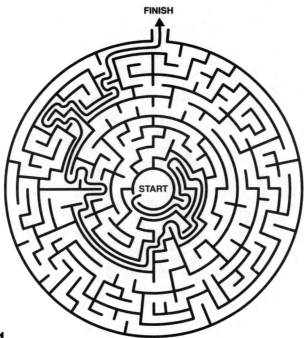

Maze 4

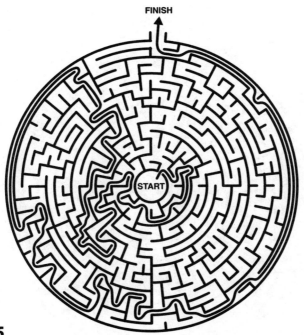

Maze 5

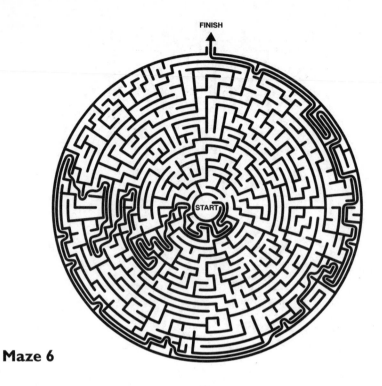

Maze 6

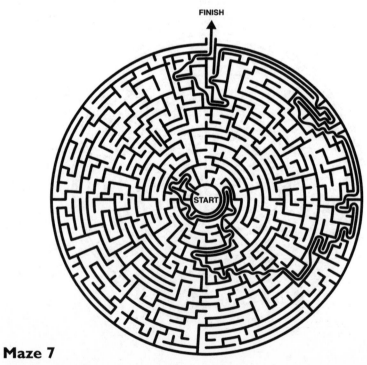

Maze 7

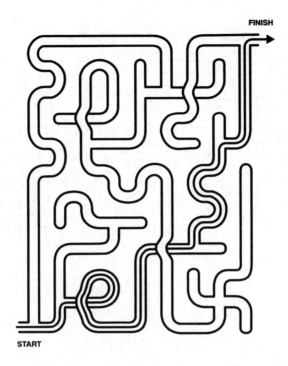

Maze 8

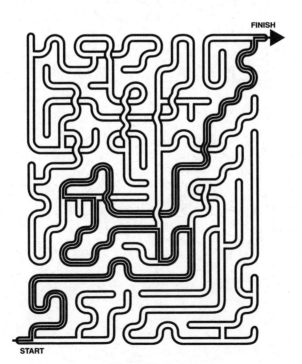

Maze 9

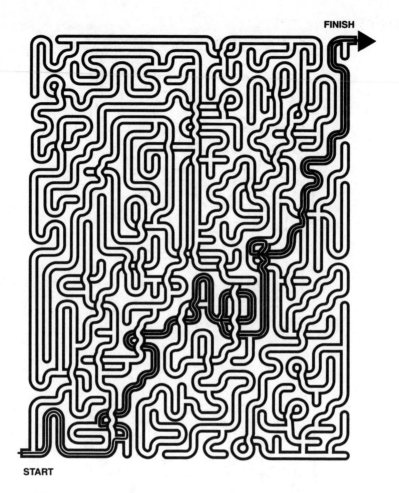

Maze 10

REFERENCES:

1. Phil Gunby, "Life Begins for Baltimore Longitudinal Study of Aging – Research Group has 40th Birthday," *Medical News & Perspectives* (April 1, 1998): 982–983.
2. K. Warner Schaie, *Intellectual Development in Adulthood* (Cambridge University Press, 1996).
3. Mathhew J. Sharps and Jana L. Sharps, "Visual Memory support: An effective mnemonic device for older adults." *Gerontologist*, 36 (5): 706–708. October 1996.
4. G.E. Finley and T. Sharp, "Name retrieval by the elderly in the Tip-of-the-Tongue paradigm: Demonstrable success in overcoming initial failure," *Educational Gerontology*, 15 (1989): 159–165.
5. Marty Munson, Theresa A Yeykal, and Susan C. Smith, "Brain Boost: Practice May Keep You Plugged," *Prevention*, 46 (1994).

E p i l o g u e

Maintain Your Brain

We hope that you have learned some new and interesting theories while reading this book. By now, you know how important the learning process is to regaining and maintaining your mental agility. The very process of reading this book has generated millions of neuron signals that passed through previously existing connections. Other millions of signals have caused the creation of new connections.

We hope you tried the various activities as you progressed through this book. You can continue to reinforce these learning and memory strategies throughout the rest of your life. Lifelong learning can take place anywhere, at any time. We recommend that you explore other materials relating to these topics. Start with the resources in the appendixes. If you were interested in some of the health issues, for example, go to the library, or go out on the Internet and research the topic. Apply the various strategies to learning about information pertinent to your lifestyle. But remember as you become comfortable with a topic or skill to stretch yourself again mentally and move on to other new and novel experiences and topics.

Let us offer one last caution. We are bombarded daily with fast, easy solutions for everything from weight loss to brain enhancement. To paraphrase Euclid, there is no royal road to mental agility. It will take critical analyses of quick-fix promotions of hormone products or other dietary supplements to determine whether they are right for you. *Always discuss products like this with your physician, even if*

they are readily available as over-the–counter supplements.
If it sounds too good to be true . . .

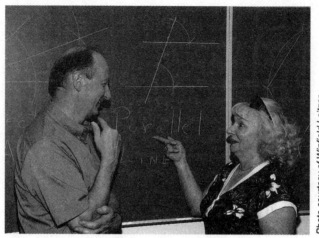

Photo courtesy of Winfield Leitzer

Older and Wiser

Dorothy Di Maio, 64, is interested in everything. *After a full career as an administrative assistant in an engineering department at a major oil company, Dorothy took early retirement at age 57. Her first reaction was* "What am I going to do with myself?"

Dorothy had always wanted to go to college, so she enrolled in the Community College of Baltimore County, Maryland. Because her job had become so automatic in the last few years, Dorothy felt that she hadn't learned much and was concerned about the challenge of college work. Dorothy took one course, German, the first semester to "see if my mind still worked." She experienced success and traveled to Germany to practice her newfound skills.

Dorothy wants to take hard *courses and is working up to taking calculus. She tries out a course to see whether she can keep up. If it gets too hard, she doesn't quit. She simply switches to audit the course and tries again for credit the next semester.*

"I'm really enjoying what I am doing," says Dorothy. She is using her brain in new and novel ways.

True mental agility is a natural outcome of natural processes. It takes hard work and consistent effort to produce results—but what remarkable results they will be!

We would like to leave you with two fundamental concepts to mull over in your newly energized mind.

Of primary importance to you are the research results that served as the basic motivation for this book. Dr. K. Warner Schaie, whose longitudinal studies focused on the effects of aging, became especially concerned with elders who, because of their mental decline, were dependent on others to care for them. His desire was to find a way to help these elders to regain enough mental ability to bring them back, or to slow the decline, so that they might live independently for a longer period of time. What he and his team found applies to all aging adults: Use your brain in new and novel ways, and you can enjoy ageless mental agility.

Second, we want you to realize that these are measures for Jane and Joe ordinary guy and gal on the street. The measures are not extraordinary. However, if you apply them daily, the cumulative effect is truly extraordinary. We're not talking about the Sophia Lorens or John Glenns of the world. We're talking about ordinary people with ordinary lives who can make their brains extraordinary simply by following the ideas in this book.

So, in summary, keep mentally and physically active. Interact with others on a daily basis. Get proper nutrition and plenty of sleep. Above all else, keep learning. Never stop learning! Every day do something to use your brain in a new and novel way, and you can enjoy ageless mental agility.

"You are never too old to set another goal or to dream a new dream." — Les Brown

A p p e n d i x

A

Annotated List of Learning Opportunities for Senior Citizens

This appendix contains a list of educational and travel opportunities you may find helpful in increasing your mental agility. Remember that the key to mental agility is to keep physically fit and to exercise your brain by learning new things.

OLDER ADULT SERVICE AND INFORMATION SYSTEM (OASIS)

Founded in St. Louis, MO, in 1982, OASIS is a national education organization designed to enhance the quality of life for mature adults. OASIS is a public-private partnership offering programs through a national network of community-based OASIS sites. Primary locations are in May Company department stores, and additional programs are offered at community sites. Members come to OASIS to attend a wide range of stimulating educational programs. Offering challenging programs in the arts, humanities, wellness, and volunteer services, OASIS creates opportunities for older adults to continue their personal growth and provide meaningful service to the community. Membership is free.

For more information, or to find the location of an OASIS center near you, contact

The OASIS Institute
7710 Carondelet Avenue
St. Louis, MO 63105
Tel: (314) 539–4555
Fax: (314) 862–2149
E-mail: OASISInst@aol.com

ELDERHOSTEL

Elderhostel is a learning program for adults 55 and older that combines inexpensive lodgings with stimulating classes on just about every subject imaginable in just about any country imaginable.

Elderhostel was founded at the University of New Hampshire as a nonprofit organization in 1975 by Marty Knowlton, a social activist and former educator, and David Bianco, a university administrator, to provide challenging educational opportunities for older adults. In the summer of 1975, five colleges and universities in New Hampshire offered the first Elderhostel programs to 220 "pioneer" hostelers. The enthusiasm was so great that when the participants were asked about their experiences, every single participant said he or she would return to Elderhostel in 1976. In 1976 more than 2,000 hostelers participated; thus began the rapid growth of Elderhostel.[1]

For questions regarding program details, enrollment, future program offerings, program availability, deposits, and so on,

- Call toll free at (877) 426–8056.
- Callers outside the U.S. and Canada: please dial (617) 426–7788.
- Hearing-impaired individuals can call toll free TTY at (877) 426–2167.

LIFELONG LEARNING IN THE USA

Most states in the U.S. have tuition abatement or reduction programs for senior citizens. In December 1991, the U.S. Senate Special Committee on Aging produced an information paper called "Lifelong Learning for an Aging Society."[1] The paper is available from the U.S. Government Printing Office. Request document ISBN 0–16–037155–4. Here is a summary of the State Survey of Statutes for Policy Concerning Tuition Fees in Higher Education Institutions conducted by the Office of Aging. This list is supplied to illustrate the general support for tuition assistance for senior citizens. Check with your local institution to learn what additional benefits have been adopted.

Alabama	There is no legislation or state policy to waive or reduce tuition for senior citizens.
Alaska	State policy waives tuition for residents 60 years or older on a space-available basis.
Arizona	There is no legislation or state policy to waive or reduce tuition for senior citizens.
Arkansas	Arkansas Code of 1987 annotated, 1989 Supp. § 6–60-Z04; § 6–51–208. Waives all general student fees at any state-supported institution of higher learning for courses organized to grant credit, and at any state area vocational-technical school, to persons 60 years or older on a space-available basis.
California	West's Annotated California Code, 1991 Supp. Education Code § 89330–§ 9333. Trustees of the California State University system may authorize the

waiver of application and regular session registration fees at any state university for enrollment in regular credit courses to persons 60 years or older, on a space-available basis.

Colorado

There is no legislation or state policy to waive or reduce tuition for senior citizens.

Connecticut

Connecticut General Statutes Annotated, 1990 Supp. § 10a—77(d)(3) Community Colleges; § 10a—83(d)(3) Community Technical Colleges. Waives tuition fee to persons 62 years or older on a space-available basis. § 10a—99(d)(3) Connecticut State University; § 10a—105(e)(3) Connecticut State University School of Medicine or Dental Medicine. Waives tuition fee for enrollment in a degree-granting program to persons 62 years or older on a space-available basis.

Delaware

Delaware Code Annotated, 1990 Supp. 14 § 3421–3422. Waives application, course, registration, and other related fees in any state-supported institution of higher learning to persons who are formal degree candidates and who are 60 years or older, on a space-available basis.

District of Columbia

The University of the District of Columbia (UDC) is the District's only state-supported school. UDC waives tuition for students 60 years or older in courses for credit or audit.

Florida

West's Florida Statutes Annotated, 1990 Supp. § 240.235(4). Waives application, course registration, and related fees in universities under the State University System, to residents who attend classes for credit and who are 60 years or older, on a space-available basis. No academic credit will be awarded under this waiver.

Georgia Official Code of Georgia, 1990 Supp. § 20–3–31.1. Waives fees (except for supplies and lab/shop fees) for courses scheduled for resident credit, except classes in dental, medical, veterinary, or law schools, to persons 62 years or older, on a space-available basis.

Hawaii Hawaii Revised Statutes Annotated, 1990 Supp. § 304–14.5. Waives tuition or fees at the University of Hawaii for any credit class to persons 60 years or older on a space-available basis.

Idaho State policy reduces registration fee to $20 plus $5 per credit hour to residents who are 60 years or older on a space-available basis. Special course fees also may be charged.

Illinois Smith-Hurd Illinois Annotated Statutes, 1990 Supp. 144 § 1801–1803. Waives tuition fee at public institutions of higher education for persons who have been accepted to enroll in regularly scheduled credit courses who are 65 years or older and whose annual household income is less than $14,000, on a space-available basis.

Indiana Burns Indiana Statutes Annotated, 1990 Supp. § 20–12–19.3–1–§ 20–12–

19.3–9. Waives 50% of tuition fee to persons 60 years or older who are retired and not working full time and who have a high school degree or equivalent, on a space-available basis. Certain other limitations are specified in § 20–12–19.3–4(c).

Iowa

There is no legislation or state policy within the university or community college system to waive or reduce tuition for senior citizens.

Kansas

State policy waives tuition at state universities for a person 60 years or older to audit courses on a space-available basis.

Kentucky

Kentucky Revised Statutes Annotated, 1990 Supp. § 164.284. Waives all tuition and fees at any state-supported institution of higher learning to any resident who is admitted and enrolled as a student and who is 65 years or older, on a space-available basis.

Louisiana

Louisiana Revised Statutes, 1991 Supp. 17:1807. Waives tuition and other registration fees at a public college or university to any person 60 years or older. Provides such persons with a 50% reduction in the cost of textbooks and other aids to instruction when purchased from a public college or university-operated bookstore. (These exemptions and reductions are provided only if sufficient funds are appropriated by the legislature to reimburse the colleges and universities affected.)

Maine

There is no legislation or state policy to waive or reduce tuition for senior citizens.

Maryland

Annotated Code of Maryland, 1990 Supp. § 13–301. Waives tuition to any constituent institution of the University of Maryland system, Morgan State University, and St. Mary's College, for up to three courses per term, to any person 60 years or older who is retired and not employed full time and whose chief income is derived from retirement benefits, on a space-available basis. (Senior citizens for whom tuition has been waived cannot exceed 2% of an institution's undergraduate full-time equivalent enrollment.) § 16–205. Waives tuition to a community college for any resident 60 years or older or for any resident who is a retired and disabled person.

Massachusetts

Massachusetts General Laws Annotated, 1990 Supp.69 § 7G. Waives tuition fees at any state college, regional community college, Southeastern Massachusetts University, Lowell University, or the University of Massachusetts for any person 60 years or older, if the institution is not overenrolled.

Michigan

Michigan Compiled Laws Annotated, 1990 Supp. § 389.123. The Board of Trustees of a community college may waive tuition for a student who meets the admission requirements of the board and who is 60 years or older.

Minnesota	Minnesota Statutes Annotated, 1991 Supp. §§ 136A.80–136A.81. Waives tuition (except for a $6 administrative fee per credit hour when taking the course for credit) and activity fee at any state university, community college, technical college, or the University of Minnesota to residents 62 years or older, on a space-available basis. The enrollee must pay laboratory and material fees.
Mississippi	There is no legislation or state policy to waive or reduce tuition for senior citizens.
Missouri	There is no legislation or state policy to waive or reduce tuition for senior citizens.
Montana	Montana Code Annotated (1989) § 20–25–421. The regents of the Montana university system may waive resident tuition to students 62 years or older. The Montana university system includes the University of Montana, Montana State University, Montana College of Mineral Science 8z Technology, Western Montana College of the University of Montana, Eastern Montana College, and Northern Montana College. § 20–25–201.
Nebraska	There is no legislation or state policy to waive or reduce tuition for senior citizens.
Nevada	State policy waives registration fee for credit or as auditors in any course to persons 62 years or older. The consent of the course instructor may be re-

quired. Such registration does not entitle a person to any privileges usually associated with registration—student association membership, health service, intercollegiate athletic tickets.

New Hampshire State policy waives only the tuition fee for persons 65 years or older on a space-available basis.

New Jersey New Jersey Statutes Annotated, 1990 Supp. 18A:62–3. Each public institution of higher education may waive tuition fees for persons 65 years or older on a space-available basis. Registration fees are not waived under this statute.

New Mexico New Mexico Statutes (1988), 1990 Supp. § 21–21D—1–§ 21–21D—5. New Mexico's postsecondary degree-granting education institutions may reduce tuition fees ($5 per credit hour, up to 6 hours per semester) to residents 65 years or older on a space-available basis. Course-specific fee charges are not waived.

New York McKinney's Consolidated Laws of New York Annotated, 1991 Supp. Education Law § 355, subd.2h(1). State-operated institutions of the state university system may waive tuition for a student who is 60 years or older to audit courses on a space-available basis.

North Carolina General Statutes of North Carolina, 1990 Supp. § 115B—1–§ 115B—6. Waives tuition at state-supported institutions of higher education, community colleges, industrial education centers, and technical institutes to attend classes for credit or noncredit, for residents 65 years or older, on a space-available basis. This waiver does not include any other fees or the cost of textbooks.

North Dakota

State policy waives tuition fees for auditing courses, for on-campus courses, to persons 65 years or older on a space-available basis.

Ohio

Ohio Revised Code Annotated (1990) § 3345.27. Waives tuition or matriculation fees at state universities or colleges for courses attended on a noncredit basis, for persons 60 years or older, on a space-available basis.

Oklahoma

State policy waives tuition fees, for auditing courses, for residents 60 years or older, on a space-available basis.

Oregon

State policy waives tuition fee to attend classes on a noncredit basis on a space-available basis.

Pennsylvania

There is no legislation or state policy to waive or reduce tuition for senior citizens.

Rhode Island

General Laws of Rhode Island, 1990 Supp. § 16–55-1. Waives tuition at any public institution of higher education to residents who are 60 years or older on a space-available basis. This benefit is at the discretion of the particular institution where application is made.

South Carolina	Code of Laws of South Carolina, 1990 Supp. § 59–111–310. Waives tuition at any state-supported college, university, or institution under the jurisdiction of the State Board for Technical and Comprehensive Education, for residents who attend credit or noncredit classes and who are 60 years or older, on a space-available basis.
South Dakota	State policy reduces tuition by one-quarter of the cost of other residents for persons 65 years or older for credit courses.
Tennessee	Tennessee Code Annotated (1990) § 49–7–113. Waives tuition, maintenance, student activity, and registration fees at state-supported colleges and universities, to persons domiciled in Tennessee, who audit courses or attend for credit and who are 65 years or older, on a space-available basis. The Board of Regents of the state university and community college system may charge a service fee not to exceed $50 a quarter or $75 a semester to defray the cost of keeping records for the student. The waiver does not apply to medical, dental, or pharmacy schools.
Texas	Texas Codes Annotated, 1991 Supp. Education Code § 54.210. The governing board of a state-supported institution of higher education may waive the tuition fee for persons 65 years or older to audit any course on a space-available basis.

Utah
Utah Code Annotated, 1990 Supp. § 53B—9–101–§ 53B—9–103. Waives tuition fees at institutions of higher learning to residents 62 years or older on a space-available basis. The quarterly registration fee is not waived.

Vermont
There is no legislation or state policy to waive or reduce tuition for senior citizens.

Virginia
Code of Virginia, 1990 Supp. § 23–38.54–§ 23–38.60. Waives tuition and registration fees at any state institution of higher education to a person who is domiciled in Virginia, who had a taxable income not exceeding $10,000 for the prior year, and who is 60 years or older, on a space-available basis. Registration is limited to no more than three courses in any one term, quarter, or semester if the person is not enrolled for academic credit, but there is no limit to the number of terms, quarters, or semesters in which a person may register.

Washington
West's Revised Code of Washington Annotated, 1991 Supp. § 28B.15.540. Boards of Regents of the state universities and State Boards for community colleges may waive tuition, service, and activity fees for a resident who is enrolled for credit (if the course credits are not used to increase credentials or salary) and who is 60 years or older, on a space-available basis. Such persons who

	enroll on an audit basis may be charged a nominal fee not to exceed $5 per quarter or semester. Registration is limited to not more than two quarter or semester courses at one time.
West Virginia	There is no legislation or state policy to waive or reduce tuition for senior citizens.
Wisconsin	West's Wisconsin Statutes Annotated, 1990 Supp. § 38–24. Waives program fees in vocational adult programs to persons 62 years or older. State policy waives tuition for all residents to audit classes within the university system.
Wyoming	There is no legislation or policy to waive or reduce tuition for senior citizens.

ADDRESSES FOR AGENCIES PROVIDING LIFELONG LEARNING OPPORTUNITIES

ALIROW
1607 Angelus Avenue
Los Angeles, California 90026

American Association of Retired Persons
601 E Street, N.W.
Washington, D.C. 20049
(202) 434–2277

Center for Creative Retirement
University of North Carolina-Asheville
Asheville, North Carolina 28804–3299
(704) 251–6140

Chemetka Community College
College for Older Adults
P.O. Box 14007
Salem, Oregon 97309
(503) 399–5139

Cherokee Nation of Oklahoma
Adult Education Program
P.O. Box 948
Tahlequah, Oklahoma 74465
(918) 456–0671, (918) 458–0484

Committee for Economic Development
477 Madison Avenue
New York, New York 10022
(212) 688–2063

Connecticut State Department on Aging
175 Main Street
Hartford, Connecticut 06106
(203) 566–4810

The Cooperative Extension Service
U.S. Department of Agriculture
Room 3444 South
14th and Independence Avenue, S.W.
Washington, D.C. 20250–0900
(202) 720–2920

Elderhostel
Elderhostel Institute Network
75 Federal Street
Boston, Massachusetts 02110–1941
(See the "Elderhostel" section, earlier in this appendix, for phone numbers.)

The External Diploma Program
The Center for Adult Learning and Educational Credentials
American Council on Education
One Dupont Circle, N.W.
Washington, D.C. 20036
(202) 939–9475

Federation of State Humanities Councils
1012 Fourteenth Street, N.W.
Suite 1007
Washington, D.C. 20005
(202) 393–5400

GED Testing Service
American Council on Education
One Dupont Circle, N.W.
Washington, D.C. 20036
(202) 939–9490

The Gerontological Society of America
1275 K Street, N.W.
Suite 350
Washington, D.C. 20005–4006
(202) 842–1275

Iowa City/Johnson County Senior Center
28 South Linn Street
Iowa City, Iowa 52240
(319) 356–5220

LaFarge Lifelong Learning Institute
1501 South Layton Boulevard
Milwaukee, Wisconsin 53215
(414) 383–2550

Lane Community College
1059 Willamette Street
Eugene, Oregon 97401–3171
(503) 726–2252

LEIF (Learning English Through Intergenerational Friendship)
Temple University
Institute on Aging
Center for Intergenerational Learning
University Services Building (083–40)
Philadelphia, Pennsylvania 19122
(215) 787–3212, (215) 787–6970

"MY TURN"
Kingsborough Community College
The City University of New York
2001 Oriental Boulevard
Brooklyn, New York 11235
(718) 368–5079

The National Council on the Aging
409 Third Street, S.W.
Suite 200
Washington, D.C. 20024
(202) 479–1200

The National Institute of Senior Centers
The National Council on the Aging, Inc.
409 Third Street, S.W.
Suite 200
Washington, D.C. 20024
(202) 479–1200

Operation ABLE of Greater Boston
World Trade Center
Suite 306
Boston, Massachusetts 02210–2078
(617) 439–5580

Poetry Program
St. Francis House Adult Day Health Care
c/o Dr. Fredda Blanchard-Fields
Department of Psychology
Louisiana State University
Baton Rouge, Louisiana 70803

Rosa Keller Campus
Touro Infirmary
The Woldenberg Center for Gerontological Studies
1401 Foucher Street
New Orleans, Louisiana 70115–3593
(504) 286–6168

Senior Multi-Purpose Center
Community Services Building
6 Gauntt Place
Flemington, New Jersey 08822
(201) 788–1359

SeniorNet
399 Arguello Boulevard
San Francisco, California 94118
(415) 750–5030

Shepherd's Centers of America
6700 Troost Street
Suite 616
Kansas City, Missouri 64131
(816) 523–1080

Siouxland Senior Center
217 Pierce Street
P.O. Box 806
Sioux City, Iowa 51102
(712) 255–1729

TESOL (Teachers of English to Speakers of Other Languages, Inc.)
1600 Cameron Street
Suite 300
Alexandria, Virginia 22314
(703) 836–0774

Union City Older Workers Day Care Training Program
138–39th Street: (201) 348–2754
219–47th Street: (201) 348–2750
Union City, New Jersey 07087

University of Massachusetts/Boston
Gerontology Program
College of Public and Community Service
Downtown Center
Boston, Massachusetts 02125
(617) 287–7330

REFERENCES:

1. www.elderhostel.org/EHORG/EHHIST.HTM
2. "Lifelong Learning for an Aging Society, Special committee on Aging, United States Senate. Serial No. 102-J. December 1991

A p p e n d i x
B

Resources for Brain Development

This appendix contains a list of books, magazines, videotapes, and other items we found helpful in increasing our mental agility. We hope you will look over the kinds of resources contained in this appendix and locate similar resources in your local libraries, agencies, and bookstores. Remember that the key to mental agility is to keep physically fit and to exercise your brain by learning new things.

BOOKS

Age Erasers for Women
Rodale Press, Inc., 1994
ISBN 0–87596–214–9
Written and compiled by the editors of Prevention Magazine Health Books and the Rodale Center for Women's Health. Provides guides and describes actions women can take to look younger and feel great. The table of contents runs from Age to Yoga and includes Longevity and Mental Health.

Fat to Firm at Any Age
by Alisa Bauman and Sari Harrar
Rodale Press, Inc., 1997
ISBN 0–87596–412–5

This book is intended as a reference only, not as a medical manual. It covers weight loss and health and hygiene of women, middle-aged women, and overweight women. Its stated purpose is to inspire and enable people to improve their lives and the world around them.

Thinking, Problem Solving, Cognition
by Richard E. Mayer
W.H. Freeman and Company, 1992
ISBN 0–7167–2214–3

Introduces the reader to the current understanding of cognition, or thinking and knowing. It has a friendly style and assumes the reader has no experience in cognitive psychology. It offers many concrete examples and illustrations. The author is a professor at the University of California, Santa Barbara.

Intellectual Development in Adulthood
by K. Warner Schaie
Cambridge University Press, 1996
ISBN 0–521–43014–3

Summarizes the results of the Seattle Longitudinal Study. Includes bibliographical references and an index. Dr. Schaie is an Evan Pugh Professor of Human Development and Psychology at Pennsylvania State University.

How the Brain Learns
by Dr. David A. Sousa
National Association of Secondary School Principals, 1995
ISBN 0–88210–301–6

This book was written for middle school and high school principals to help train their teachers in the latest brain research. Because you are interested in lifelong learning, this book will help you by knowing how teachers are using the new results and how you might use them to continue your learning. According to Dr. Sousa, effective learning makes the best use possible of experience, attention span, memory/recall patterns, right/left orientation, and practice. For information, contact

The National Association of Secondary School
Principals
1904 Association Drive
Reston, VA 22091–1537
Tel: (703) 860–0200
Fax: (703) 476–5432

PERIODICALS

AARP Bulletin
The American Association of Retired Persons
ISSN 1044–1123

Covers areas of concern such as Medicare and Social Security. Typical topics include medical frauds, telephone frauds, the reassessment of seniors' driving, and new techniques in treating diseases that affect the elderly.

This bulletin is published monthly, except in August. For information, contact

The American Association of Retired Persons
601 E. Street, N.W.
Washington, D.C. 20049

The Brain in the News
edited by Randy Talley
The Dana Press

A recent issue discussed proof of the regeneration of brain cells in adult humans, as well as the study of children's brains when they were reading silently and aloud.

You can obtain a free subscription to this fine newsletter by contacting

Randy Talley
The Dana Press
1001 G St. N.W., Suite 1025
Washington, D.C. 20001
Tel: (202) 737–9200
E-mail: rtalley@dana.org

BRAIN WORK, the Neuroscience Newsletter
The Charles A. Dana Foundation
This is a bimonthly publication that chronicles developments in brain research. You can contact The Charles A. Dana Foundation at

The Charles A. Dana Foundation
745 Fifth Avenue, Suite 700
New York, NY 10151

Dell Crossword Puzzles
Dell Magazines
This magazine is published monthly and contains many types of challenging crossword puzzles. It also lists puzzle magazines and their publishing dates. Dell Crossword Puzzles are available at newsstands or by single copy at

Dell Magazines
1540 Broadway
New York, New York 10036

Games Magazine
Games Publications, Inc.
Known as "the magazine for creative minds at play." Among the games are crossword and crossnumber puzzles, a variety of pencil puzzles, cryptograms, eyeball benders, and many others. This challenging and exciting magazine is published bimonthly by

Games Publications, Inc.
P.O. Box 2031
Marion, OH 43305–2031
Tel: (800) 426–3768

Life **magazine**
July 1994

This issue is probably available at your local library. It includes several articles, such as "Building a Better Brain," p. 62, that you will enjoy reading.

VIDEOTAPES

Ancient Secret of the Fountain of Youth, The Video
Harbor Press, Inc., 1999
ISBN 0–936197–33–1

This exercise tape provides a low-stress exercise workout. Sections include

    Reverse the Telltale Signs of Aging
    Lose Weight and Look Great
    Become Firm, Fit and Fantastic
    Feel Energetic, Alive and Lively
    Eliminate Stress and Melt Away Tension
    Enjoy Total Health and Wellness

You can contact Harbor Press at

Harbor Press, Inc.
P.O. Box 1656
Gig Harbor WA 98335

YOGA Practice
Healing Arts Publishing, Inc., 1996
ISBN 0–945671–81–4

This is a set of six videotapes for learning the basics of yoga. Sections include

    Practice for Beginners
    Practice for Flexibility

Practice for Strength
Practice for Relaxation
Practice for Meditation
Practice for Energy

CATALOGS

Bits & Pieces, The Source for Puzzles and Gifts

To request a free catalog, call (800)-JIGSAWS (800–544–7279) or go online at www.bitsandpieces.com.

Critical Thinking Books & Software

To request a free 61-page catalog, call (800) 458–4849.

GAMES Direct, Games and Puzzles for Teens & Grown-ups

To request a free 32-page catalog, call (800) 344–3328.

Organized Thinking, Exercise Equipment for the Brain

For a brochure, write to

220 Boylston Street, Suite 306
Newton, MA 02167

Smart Games, Inc.

This is a software company that specializes in brain games. It runs a gaming league over the Internet. Visit www.smartgames.com to learn more, or write to

Smart Games, Inc.
49 Atlantic Avenue
Marblehead, MA 01945

SCREENING TESTS

Depression Screening Tests

For those who may be experiencing depression or know someone who is, Ann Landers has set up a toll-free number to tell you the names and numbers of the depression screening centers closest to you. This is an automated message, so it is completely anonymous. Call (800) 242–2211. TTY for the hearing impaired is (800) 855–2880.

Olfactory Test

An easy, self-administered test is the University Of Pennsylvania Smell Identification Test. It identifies impairment in the sense of smell and is available from

Sensonics, Inc.
125 White Horse Pike
Haddon Heights, NJ 08035
Tel: (609) 547–7702

Appendix
C

Using the Web for Lifelong Learning

The World Wide Web is a breakthrough in technology that gives people the opportunity to communicate quickly, learn new things, and find information rapidly. Basically, it is a clever, easy way to use the Internet to get information with a minimum of fuss. What we need to know to begin using it is very little. It's really a vocabulary lesson when we get right down to it. In the next few paragraphs, we will define the terms you may or may not have heard relating to the World Wide Web, or WWW, for short. You then will be able to use "old" technology, the telephone, to order what you need to get up and running on the Web.

But first, let's talk about a good reason why this appendix is in a book on new learning techniques. The ability to learn new things is pretty useless without resources to help you learn what you want to know more about. The Internet is chock full of new information. But if you can't access it, what good is it? This appendix will help you learn the basics so that you can acquire the resources you need to begin learning what is on the Internet.

One of the organizations that helps is the SeniorNet. Before you think that this is an organization simply for older people, you should know that SeniorNet is a nonprofit group that helps bring technology to all people over the age of 30. The number of seniors who have access to the Internet rose from 17 percent in 1995 to a whopping 75 percent in 1998, says Eileen Colkin, a contributing author to *Information Week.*[1]

Here are some other interesting numbers Eileen reported:

- 15 percent of seniors classify themselves as heavy users (more than 10 hours online per week).
- 70 percent use electronic mail, or e-mail.
- 40 percent check out hobby- or health-related sites.
- 38 percent visit investment sites.

The difference between the WWW and the Internet is a bit blurred. The WWW is a part of the Internet. When you use a computer program called a *browser,* you are viewing "pages" on the Web. Other activities occur on the Internet, but we generally use the WWW to access free information. The Internet is the collection of individual computer networks all over the world that exchange information. The WWW is the collection of computers (Web servers) that provide specially formatted pages for people using a browser. Examples of browsers are Netscape Navigator™, Microsoft's Internet Explorer™, and America Online's™ (AOL's) user programs.

If you want to access the information on all of these computers all over the world, you need to have *Internet service.* A company that connects your computer to the Internet is called an *Internet service provider* (ISP). Samples of these are America Online, Erols, Compuserve, @Home, *Microsoft Network* (MSN), and many, many others. Each provider charges a bit differently for its service to you. So, you need a computer and an ISP. The ISP provides the browser for your use.

You also need a modem and a mouse. A *modem* connects your computer to the ISP and then to the Internet through your telephone line. In some areas, your local cable company offers a high-speed modem that connects you to the Internet via fiber-optic cable. A *mouse* is a device that enables you to perform a number of operations on the computer without having to type a great deal on the computer's keyboard. This is a bonus for those of us who are still one-finger typists!

Using a browser is quite easy, once you get the hang of it. It communicates with the other computers on the Web to locate information for you. The information is organized into collections of Web pages located all around the world. These collections are called *Web sites*. Each Web page has a unique identifier—a name, if you like. This is called its *uniform resource locator*, or *URL*. You can't miss URLs in our culture today. You see them at the bottom of the TV screen in advertisements, in magazines, on vehicles, on billboards—just about everywhere. They generally start out with these three lowercase letters: www. For example, the Web site associated with this text is www.mentalagility.com. If you know the address of a page, you can type it into your browser, and the Web finds the page you want and displays it on your computer. This process is called *downloading*.

After you find a page you are interested in, you will find blue highlighted and/or underlined words or phrases. These are called *hyperlinks,* or *links* for short. After you click on one of these links with your mouse, you get another Web page to look at without having to type in the URL. When you are moving around the Internet by clicking links, you are said to be *surfing the Net*.

If you don't know the address of a specific page, but you know what you are looking for by name, you can use a *search engine*. This is special type of Web page that locates other Web pages for you.

Examples of search engines are www.altavista.com, www.yahoo.com, and www.snap.com. An easy search engine to use is AskJeeves. This site accepts English sentences and searches for what you want. For example, you might want to ask "How many senior citizens have computers?" Visit www.AskJeeves.com and type in your question. Jeeves will provide a list of Web sites to visit to answer that question. See Figure C-1.

Most people join the Internet for one reason: e-mail. It's

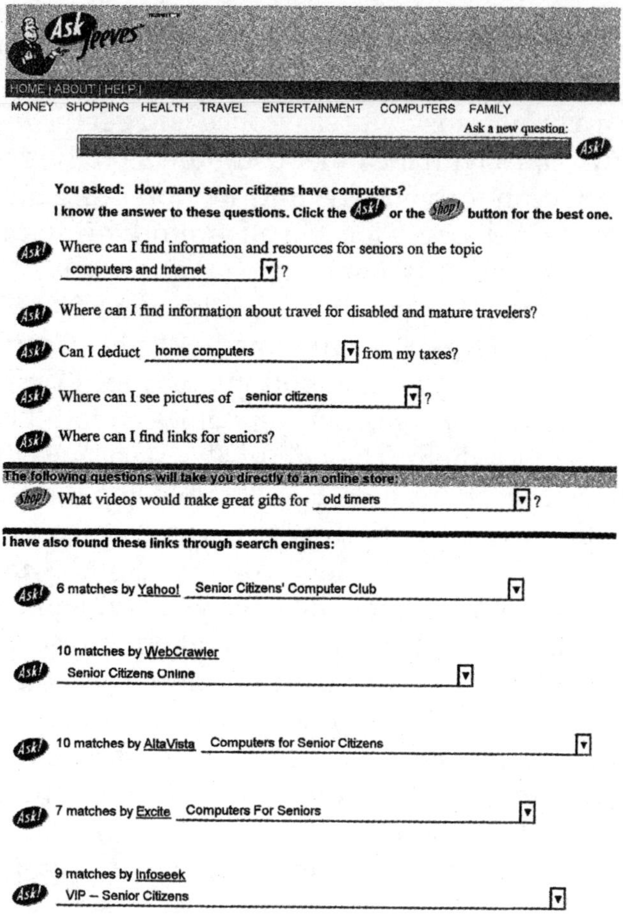

Figure C-1 © Ask Jeeves, Inc. 1999. All rights reserved. Reprinted with Permission.

the rage of the decade. Electronic mail consists of messages you type into the computer and send to anyone who also has an e-mail account. Usually, you get an e-mail account included with your Internet service. There are also free e-mail accounts, provided by several Web pages that show advertisements.

You can identify an e-mail address by its characteristic structure. At the front of an e-mail address is a person or a code for a person's name. In the middle is the @ sign. At the end is the name of service provider, or the name of the

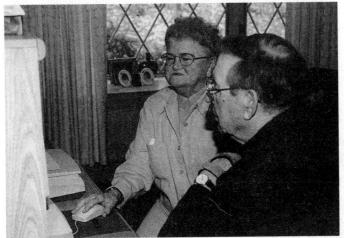

Photo courtesy of Winfield Leitzer

Learning New Tricks

*Chuck and Jacque Gibson bought a new computer (their second)
to help them in their bookkeeping business. They are having the time
of their lives learning a new trick: scanning photographs and ex-
changing them via e-mail with their children and grandchildren.*

computer where an electronic mailbox exists. A sample is
`kcwetzel@mentalagility.com` or `information@
mentalagility.com`.

Many people are finding it fun and easy to send photos
attached to an e-mail message. They have a device attached
to their computers called a *scanner*. A scanner copies a physical photograph into an electronic version that can be sent
across the Internet and viewed at another computer.

You can access other features on the Internet with an ISP.
There are archives of conversations on myriad topics, called
newsgroups. There are discussion groups you can join to exchange e-mail messages, called *mailing lists*. You also can *download* computer programs. This means that if software is
available on another computer, you can copy it to your computer. This type of software can be licensed, shareware, or free-

ware. *Shareware* means that you can try the software before you pay for it. And generally, the price is very small if you do decide to keep the software. And, you can type in a message in a live conversation with other people using the Internet. This activity is called *chat*.

Whatever you decide to use the Internet for, you will learn new things, feel connected to the world, exercise old connections, and create new connections as you learn how to use the Internet.

In this appendix, we have collected a list of interesting sites for you to visit as you learn how to use the Internet. A word of caution, though: The Internet is a dynamic place. New pages are posted daily, and old ones are removed. Some people move their Web pages around. The problem is that an address may have changed. If the browser cannot locate a page you specify, try typing the simple Web site name without all of the extra parts of the address. For example, there is a wonderful card trick puzzle on this page: www3. mcps.k12.md.us/users/rsfay/magic. However, the owner, Montgomery County Public Schools in Maryland, may choose to move it around in the future. Try typing in just the first half of the address: www3.mcps.k.12.md.us and surfing to find the card trick.

As an assistance, the authors will keep an up-to-date list of these addresses that you can check out on www. mentalagility.com. *Do not call the publisher!* They will not be able to help you with this situation. Please note that because Internet resources are of a time-sensitive nature and URL addresses may change or be deleted, searches should also be conducted by association and/or topic.

Try These Fun and Interesting Web Sites

www.puzzlemaker.com supplies a cutout puzzle and logo.

www.puz.com offers free software to download from puzzler Russell Sasamori.

For e-commerce and to find out about books for sale, try www.borders.com or www.barnesandnoble.com

`www.newswise.com` gives you late-breaking news and press releases.

`www.med.nyu.edu/Psych/screens` provides an online depression screening test.

`www.mindtools.com/mnemlsty.html` tells you how learning styles affect your use of mnemonics.

`www.wordsmith.org` has lots of wonderful activities available, including an anagram generator. Type a word or phrase, say, your name, and the site generates anagrams for you. Also, you can join a mailing list that sends you a word a day. Your vocabulary will grow by leaps and bounds.

`www.alz.org` tells you more about the Alzheimer's Association.

`www.aoa.dhhs.gov/aoa/pages/jpostlst.html` provides an *Online Directory on Internet and E-mail Resources on Aging*.

`www.pbs.org` provides information about brain works and technology changes in the home.

`www.seniornet.org` lists locations throughout the U.S. where seniors can get computer training.

`www.seniorhousing.net` lets you search a directory of retirement communities, assisted-living facilities, and nursing homes for you or your loved ones. You can access a glossary of terms you'll need to know if you are looking into new housing.

`intp.org/test.html` (Some Web sites do not begin with www, but they behave the same way.) Look for a page listing "A Plethora of Tests." Here you can find out more about your personality, take an IQ test, and more.

`www.2h.com/Tests/iqtrad.phtml` gives you many more tests.

www.brainergy.com is a site for cerebral fitness training for the adult brain.

www.census.gov provides access to the national census (general data).

www.aarp.org is the address for the American Association of Retired Persons.

www.oww.com is a site called *Older, Wiser & Wired: A Virtual Community for Netsurfers Over 50.*

www.realage.com is a site that checks up on a variety of life-lengthening activities.

www.dejanews.com helps you find newsgroups.

www.elderhostel.com provides information on the Elderhostel, including how to register and what courses are available in their catalogs.

www.refdesk.com/paper.html is a URL that not only links to newspapers worldwide, but is also a reference desk. You can find links to a thesaurus, calculator, almanac, and much, much more.

A site that allows you to create puzzles and games is available at www.puzzlemaker.com

Find out about recent results in sleep research at www.sleepfoundation.org

These are only a sampling of the pages available for increasing your mental agility. After you get out there on the Web, you will find many more. Share them with us at www.mentalagility.com

Happy surfing and productive searching!

REFERENCES:

1. "Surfin' Seniors," Information Week (October 26, 1998).

Index

A

Accommodation, combatting mental decline, 211
Acetylcholine, memory maintenance, 175
Adaptability, fighting stress, 190
Addresses, e-mail, 326
Adults, brain development, 28
Aerobic exercise, 180-181
Ageless mental agility, 207-208
Agencies for life-long learning, 309
Agility of mind, 208
Aging
  affects of process, self-quiz, 149
  Aging process quiz, 125-126
  cognitive aspects, 146-147
  cross-sectional studies, 126
  longitudinal studies, 127
  physical aspects, 129
  hearing, 132-135
  perceptual window, 131
  reaction time, 142-144
  retrieval time, 142-144
  skeleton, 141
  sleep patterns, 142
  smell, 138-139
  taste, 138
  touch, 139
  vision, 129-130
  psychological aspects, 144-145
  slowing process
    balanced diet, 178
    exercise, 179-181, 187
    fighting stress, 189-190
    massage therapy, 191
    personal techniques, 154-156, 161-162
    positive creative outlook, 189
    proper nutrition, 173, 178
    proper sleep, 165, 170
    resetting biological clock, 159

J-K

L